THE BELLY AND ITS POWER

plus seven other articles on the restoration of
health, balance and vitality

by Allan Saltzman

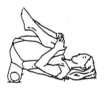

YOGA TOOLS INC.
P.O. Box 3286
New Haven, CT 06515

ISBN 0-941821-00-5

Library of Congress Card Number 87-050038

Yoga Tools Inc.
P.O. Box 3286
New Haven, CT 06515

Printed in the United States

Fourth Printing

*To my wife Janice
without whose support
and inspiration this
book would not have
been written*

CONTENTS

INTRODUCTION

These essays and articles were written over an eight year period. They are an expression of and a glimpse of an important biological process. This is a healing process but also one of growth and personal evolution. Central to this process is the development of that inner body sense called kinesthesia. If the condition of our muscles, joints, organs and blood vessels can become conscious to us through this inner and subtle sense, we will naturally be inclined toward this healing process. This healing process is a lesson or a series of lessons in rest and relaxation. It is a surrender and a letting go at the very deepest physical levels and all that can mean.

Each one of these eight articles is a glimpse or a snapshot of that process, trying to capture in words and pictures something of its nature and meaning. Being a glimpse it is necessarily incomplete. I'm sure a book could be devoted to each subject and I know many that already have. I didn't set out to write a book and so each article has a finality about it that I have only slightly altered to fit into a book format.

What holds these essays together is that they are all about a natural healing process of relaxation and release. They are my attempt at understanding that process and to express as succinctly as possible some of its major features.

THE BELLY AND ITS POWER

The Liberation of the Natural Energy Center in Man

Illustrated
by
David Davis
Linda McKone

1

THE BELLY AND ITS POWER

"Belly in, chest up, shoulders back." This, we are told, represents good posture and good looks. America wants to "tighten its gut" because the flat, hard stomach is considered one of the cornerstones of physical fitness. To have any sign of a belly protruding makes us fat and lazy, in need of doing sit-ups and leg raisers to "tone" those lazy stomach muscles. The man with the fifty inch chest and thirty inch waist becomes Mr. America and represents the body beautiful. With a round, full belly we are considered to be either pregnant or heavy beer drinkers. Now even a best-selling book appears with the title *How to Flatten Your Stomach*.

Much of the world disagrees. The Japanese word hara literally means belly. Hara Kiri means belly splitting, the warrior's style of suicide, where the abdomen is cut and the viscera spill out. To the Japanese, cutting the hara is attacking life at its source, the belly.

Karlfried Durkheim's book *Hara, The Vital Centre of Man* is a serious and scholarly look at the whole range of the hara concept in the culture of Japan. "Hara", he writes, "implies for the Japanese all that he considers essential to man's character and destiny. Hara is the centre of the human body ... It is at the same time the centre in a spiritual sense or, to be more accurate, a nature given spiritual sense." [1]

The man with belly is centered, tranquil, balanced. He is "large minded, one who is magnanimous and warm hearted". [2]

Conversely, the man without a belly lacks calm judgement. He reacts haphazardly and capriciously. He is easily

2

startled and nervous ... he lacks that inner axis which would prevent his being thrown off center. "The man with no belly is in every respect a picture of immaturity."[3]
    Traditionally then for the Japanese, hara, the belly, has meant strength, maturity and a tranquil mind.

CENTER OF GRAVITY

With our prejudice against the belly we tend to see strength in big arms and broad shoulders. We feel a belly detracts from this image of strength. Mental power derives from our head, our brain specifically. We locate physical and mental power well above our navels.
    Al Huang in the book *Embrace Tiger, Return to Mountain* describes the difference between the Oriental and the Western man:
"The Oriental man is very empty and light up here in the head and very heavy down here in the belly and he feels very secure. The Western man is light in the belly and very heavy up here in the head, so he topples over."[4]
    In the practice of Tai Chi and other oriental martial arts the center of gravity is located in the lower belly and the reservoir of Life Energy or Breath Energy is also in the lower belly. From this "single spot in the lower abdomen"[5] movement begins and energy is made. This spot is revered as the source of life in man. In Chinese yoga it is pictured as a burning cauldron producing the energy needed to open up and liberate the rest of the body.

BREATHING

The anatomical facts give support to the Oriental viewpoint. The diaphragm is a broad, flat, dome-shaped muscle that separates the thoracic (chest) cavity from the abdominal cavity. The diaphragm is our principle breathing muscle; its use is crucial for breathing deeply. Unfortunately, in the majority of people, tension in and around the abdominal region so restricts diaphragmatic breathing that the resulting capacity to breathe is possibly one-third to one-quarter of what it should be.

When used, this dome-shaped muscle contracts and flattens out, pushing down upon the contents of the abdomen. With this pressure exerted from above by the action of the diaphragm, the abdominal region, particularly the soft front wall, expands. This ability to expand or blow up the belly with an inhalation is the outward sign that the diaphragm is functioning.

Very simply, the body must be able to expand and contract to breathe. Limitations on our ability to do this restricts our capacity to breathe. Using the belly is not in itself a full breath. The flexibility and action available in the rib cage further increases the breath capacity. The total and complete breath first appears to fill up the abdomen; the belly noticeably expands like a balloon. Finally the expanding impulse moves through the entire rib cage to the top of the chest. The action is fluid and wave-like, beginning low in the belly and rising to the top of the chest. In the process, the entire trunk of the body expands. A full exhalation involves the lowering of the chest and a contraction of the belly.

Anyone familiar with the experience of complete breathing knows that it is predominently a sensation of filling and blowing up the abdomen. Here in the soft and flexible abdominal wall, the body has its greatest potential to expand. The ribs themselves offer limited movement. The belly is really the bellows that fills us up.

Of course, air does not fill up the belly. The abdominal contents are merely responding to a downward physical pressure exerted by the diaphragm muscle. This creates a partial vacuum in the lungs which draws air in from the outside.

Now if the muscles of the body, particularly those surrounding the abdominal region, are held too tightly, a deep breath will be impossible, and yet, inelastic, hard muscles in the abdomen are the kind of muscles most stomach exercises are designed to create.

A healthy mid-section is surprisingly soft and flexible. It gives easily during breathing and allows the internal organs of digestion and elimination the space they need to function properly. Maintain a constriction in the abdominal muscles and not only do you choke off breathing but the vital internal organs are compressed and distorted. Life is literally strangled.

BREATH ENERGY

Little has been said or written on the energy and endurance produced by simply opening up the breathing. Much has appeared on how running or swimming eventually improves physical endurance but the real key to physical power is not how many miles you run in a day, but how well you breathe. Learn to breathe fully and endurance is yours forever, whenever you want it.

Beyond the endurance that comes with opened breathing

is an impetus towards personal evolution. Though shrouded in mystery and myth, Chinese and Indian yoga point towards a real process that alters the basic structure of our bodies and our minds. In Indian yoga this evolutionary power or impulse is called prana; in China, chi; in Japan, ki. Here is an energy that streams through the body and on which our health depends. Block this energy and we become ill.

In every case this internal force is related to breathing. Open the breathing up, especially deep into the belly, and the body becomes charged with energy. This is the energy that drives us towards wholeness and perfection. In a very real sense, an opened capacity to breathe is only the first step in the evolution to which the various yogas refer. Breathing creates the awareness, the force and the drive out of which comes the earnest practice of yoga.

LIFE FORCE

As the breathing deepens and the body learns to relax, the awareness is increasingly drawn to a point down in the pit of the belly. With relaxation consciousness spends less time in the head and more time just naturally attracted to the heart area or to the pit of the belly. This spot beneath the navel and in the pit of the belly is not just some abstract point in space but the charged and energized center of the human being. Here lies the source of sexual energy and excitement but also a potential impulse towards health, openness and freedom.

Learn to let go and relax and the mind is drawn to the source of life. Consciousness and the Life Force are united in the pit of the belly.

THE NATURAL CHILD

In our midst are people who are living and shining examples of what a relaxed belly and a capacity to fully breathe can mean. These people are our children. The bellies of our two and three year olds are not flat or hard yet. The power of their naturalness has not been seriously restrained so their bellies bulge and they breathe well. Young children glow and overflow with energy. They delight us with their spontaneity and playfulness. They usually seem happy or at least have a tremendous capacity for pleasure and enjoyment. We either ignore their curious physical condition (those ballooning bellies) or explain it as immature structure that will change.

Western civilization has pictured man as flatbellied for thousands of years. We have used our heads and our hands to create science, technology, and great material comfort and wealth. The time may be nearing when we will need to loosen our bellies, breathe easily again, and so enjoy what we have created.

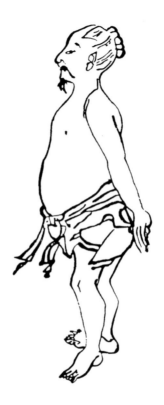

THE MAN WITH BELLY

The three drawings of oriental men in this book are taken from acupuncture diagrams that are thousands of years old. We can see that the ancient Chinese had an image of man with a definite belly, and yet these are not men who are weak or sick. Their apparent sturdiness and strength is built around their bellies. Their center of gravity is low and they appear stable and well-rooted to the ground. These are mature and relaxed men who can breathe deeply and well.

THE LIBERATION OF THE NATURAL ENERGY CENTER IN MAN

THE ILIOPSOAS MUSCLE

A common misconception about protruding bellies is that they are a product of weak abdominal muscles. By this reasoning the abdominal muscles are weak and soft so the contents of the abdomen push out and thereby put a strain on the lower back. We end up with a posture that has a protruding belly and a swayback condition called a lordosis.

A growing knowledge and appreciation of body mechanics is showing the inaccuracy of this reasoning. The real key to good posture is not the abdominal muscles but the iliopsoas muscle. The iliopsoas is a broad, powerful muscle that attaches on the upper inside of the pelvic basin and lower spine (lumbar), traverses over the pelvic basin and attaches to the upper inside section of the thigh bone (femur). The function of the iliopsoas is to flex the leg upon the trunk of the body as when the leg swings forward in walking. The iliopsoas muscle is also crucial in determining the amount of tilt the pelvis takes. A tight iliopsoas muscle tends to compress the lumbar spine towards the groin. The lower back and the groin area are stressed by a short, tight iliopsoas and eventually will distort out of their proper position. The pelvis will assume a forward tilt creating that characteristic swayback condition and an excessively protruding belly.

Doing thirty sit-ups a day to tighten and flatten the abdominal region is often not only futile but harmful. The sit-ups will only add further stress and tension to the tightened iliopsoas muscle, the real cause of the postural problem.

The best solution is to stretch and lengthen the iliopsoas muscle. When the iliopsoas assumes its natural length and span, the posture will tend to correct itself. No amount of effort in standing straight and holding the stomach in can ever succeed in improving posture. When the stress in the iliopsoas is relieved, gravity itself will align and straighten the body. Good posture then can come easily and naturally.

**THE
ILIOPSOAS
MUSCLE**

PSOAS MAJOR

ILIACUS

STRETCHING THE ILIOPSOAS

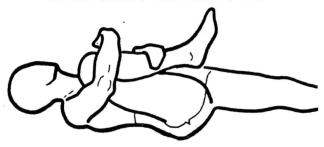

This is the most common exercise recommended by orthopedic doctors. With the body flat on the floor one leg is brought up and gently pulled against the chest. The greater the difficulty in doing this exercise the tighter the iliopsoas muscle is. If the leg resting upon the floor rises up too much this indicates a shortened iliopsoas.

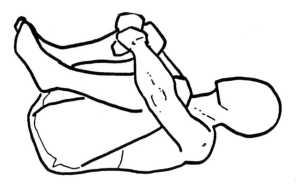

Pulling both knees to the chest offers a moderate traction and stretch for the lower back. This may also be felt into the groin area indicating that the iliopsoas' lower connection (upon the upper inside section of the thigh bone) is being stretched.

LEG SPREADS FOR THE ILIOPSOAS

Much of the strain of a shortened iliopsoas is felt in the groin. Tension and shortened muscles in this area inevitably reflect some sexual problem. Opening and stretching the groin area is difficult but important.

Stretch slowly and gently without subjecting yourself to more pain than you can easily tolerate. When bringing the legs together after stretching them apart, feel for any vibration or quivering movements in the hips. Let yourself vibrate if you can for as long as possible. Involuntary vibrations mean the muscles are beginning to loosen and release the energy stored in tension.

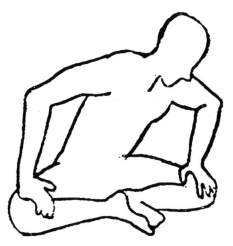

Sitting on the floor put your feet together and draw them in towards the groin. Sitting up as straight as possible apply pressure with the hands to the knees. The tighter the hips are the further the knees will be from the floor. This posture is also a Natural Childbirth exercise designed to give a more open and flexible quality to the pelvis.

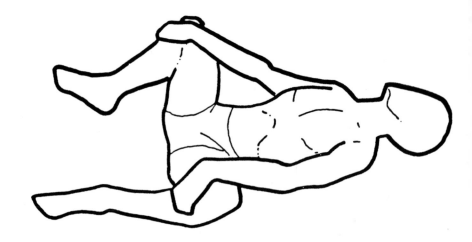

Lying flat on the floor bring the knees up and grasp them on the inside with your hands. Let the legs spread apart by their own weight. The arms are held straight while gravity does the work in this stretch. If needed, this stretch should be felt strongly into the groin. From this position still grasping the inside of the knees pull up on them slightly, one knee or both knees at a time. This will stretch further into the groin.

After a series of stretches for the hips and groin, it is usually a good idea to stand up and move the hips around in circles. Feel for rough, stiff areas in the hip joints as they rotate and move around. Mobilizing this lower segment of the body with this simple fluid exercise lubricates the hip joints, relieves some of the stress in the muscles previously stretched, and eventually will stimulate and deepen the breathing.

ABDOMINAL SELF-MASSAGE

It seems like the whole country is trying to tighten and harden its stomach, a very misdirected effort. This section is about doing just the opposite. The object of self-massage is to soften and loosen what is hard and stiff, to create a condition of suppleness and flexibility.

Softness is not the same thing as weakness. This is a difficult concept to accept, but for muscles it is true. A hard muscle is in a state of contraction; a soft muscle is relaxed. A relaxed muscle can be hardened instantly by contracting it, but by maintaining that contraction in the muscle it will eventually fatigue and weaken. A soft muscle is ready for action; a hard muscle is already hard at work and near fatigue. A soft muscle will work longer than one that is hard.

Soft muscles feel liquid. A relaxed abdomen is soft to the touch. The fingers can penetrate into the intestines and colon without meeting resistance from the muscles. There is no pain or sensitivity when the fingers probe into the deeper viscera.

Abdominal regions that are soft and yielding are the exception though. Most bellies, even the bigger ones, are not soft. The probing fingers meet a wall of tension and resistance. Areas of pain and sensitivity are everywhere.

Abdominal self-massage is a very direct way to improve one's health and to become aware of the body's core condition.

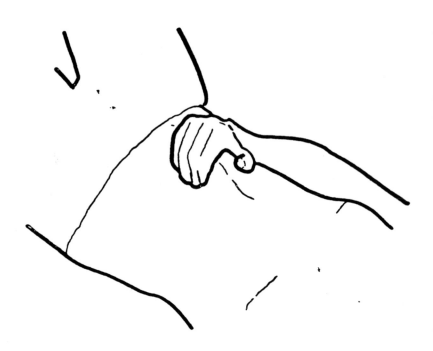

Lying on your back bend the legs so the knees are off the floor and the feet flat on the floor. With the legs bent up like this the stomach muscles tend to be more relaxed.

Take a big handful of abdominal tissue beneath the navel. Move it around in circles, press it in and out and generally stimulate and vibrate the area. The tighter the region the more resistance there will be. When relaxed the tissue should feel soft and supple and will ripple and wave almost like water.

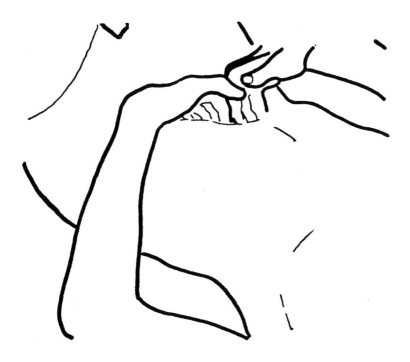

Probing in deeper with the fingers feel for areas of pain and sensitivity. These sensitive areas can often be felt in the colon or up underneath the ribs on either side. Where there is spasticity in the colon there will be tenderness, and pain up under the ribs suggests stomach, gall bladder, or liver problems.

Abdominal massage can give you an early warning signal of impending trouble. Most problems begin as tension and stiffness and to deal with these problems at that level is good preventive medicine.

THE SQUAT

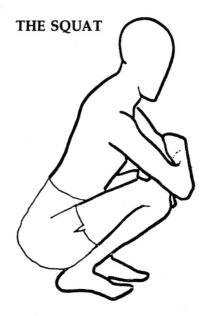

Squatting is a perfectly natural position. Children assume the position easily in the course of play and most primitive peoples sit in the squat for long periods of time. Because of our complete reliance on furniture, squatting is difficult and foreign for many of us.

The simple squatting position has the feet slightly apart and the heels on the ground. If this is too difficult place a cushion or rolled towel underneath the heels.

Squatting is the natural position for moving the bowels. The squat tends to stretch open the anus while the thighs press into the abdominal area aiding the movement of feces.

Sitting in the squatting position for a few minutes or more gives the legs, the hips and lower back a gentle stretch. The entire lower half of the body is stimulated with increased circulation.

STRETCHING THE ABDOMINAL MUSCLES

Most stomach muscles are not weak. If a person can do one sit-up, his or her muscles are strong enough. Sitting up is a good test of stomach muscle strength but not a good general exercise because of the strain it usually places on the hips and back.

Time would be better spent on stretching and lengthening the abdominal muscles. As the abdominal area opens and stretches, the breathing impulse can fill the belly and allow for deeper, fuller breathing.

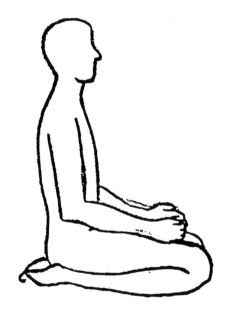

This is the traditional Japanese sitting posture. Sitting on the heels, the feet and the front of the legs and thighs are stretched. Place a cushion beneath the ankles and on top of the heels to relieve knee strain if necessary.

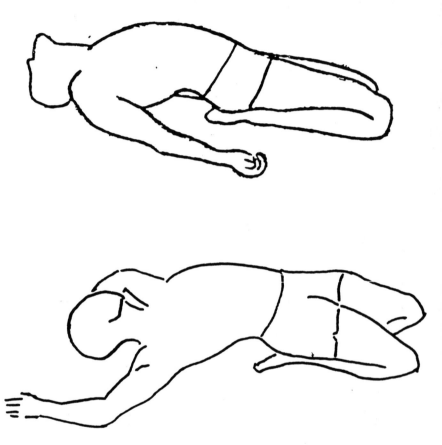

Starting from the Japanese sitting posture, lean very slowly back first onto the hands placed behind the body and then onto the elbows, top of the head, and then finally to the shoulders on the floor. At each step different muscle groups will be stretched. This is a difficult posture that may take many months to completely master. Eventually when the shoulders are on the floor and with the arms extended up over the head, the entire abdominal region is stretched and expanded.

USING A ROLLER TO EXPAND THE HIPS AND CHEST AND TO STRETCH THE ABDOMEN

Use a Spinal Roller* or a rolling pin rolled up as tightly as possible with one or two folded towels and then secured with elastics or string.

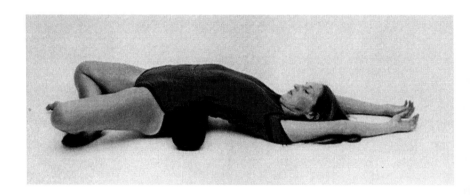

To stretch the iliopsoas and other deep hip muscle that control pelvic tilt and posture, put the roller underneath the sacrum. The feet are together and drawn in towards the body. The knees fall out by their own weight. If this stretch is needed it will be felt in the groin and into the hips. Move the roller down to the coccyx or up to the lumbar section of the spine to stretch the whole range of muscles in the hips. Extend and stretch the arms over the head which will lift the rib cage and stretch the muscles of the abdomen.

*For more information on the Spinal Roller write to: Yoga Tools, P.O. Box 3286, New Haven, CT, 06515.

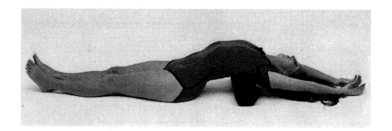

Bend backwards over the roller placed beneath the shoulder blades. Again stretch the arms up over the head to lift the ribs. The chest is stretched and opened and so is the diaphragm muscle.

Try holding both positions for a minute or more for maximum benefit. See if the breathing starts to deepen naturally as the diaphragm opens and the abdomen stretches and expands.

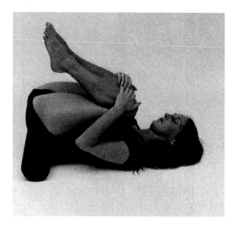

Place the roller under the lower part of the back and pull the knees up towards the chest. This stretches and opens the lumbar spine.

SPINAL STRETCHES AND SPINAL ROLLING

At some point in the process of releasing deeper energies and expanding physical awareness, the spine becomes our principle focus. It dawns on us that the back is stiff and tense. Some areas may be worse than others but the whole spine is affected.

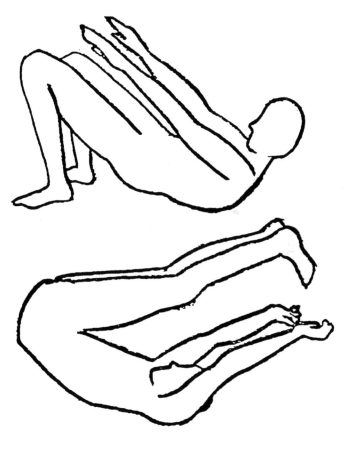

Using a thinly carpeted section of floor with possibly only a blanket added as cushion, the back and spine can be massaged and rolled. The hardness and firmness of the floor is important and should be felt and used to press into and massage over stiff, tight areas. The back may even crunch and snap as these areas of stiffness are worked out. Spinal curvatures and distortions may be sensed and these too can be rolled and smoothed out over the course of some months doing these maneuvers.

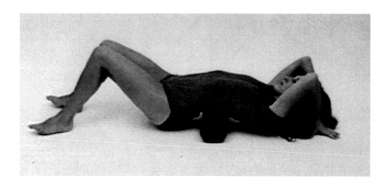

Roll and press the spinal roller along the entire length of the spine. The spinal roller adds a more penetrating dimension to spinal rolling maneuvers. Different areas of the back relate to internal organ function. By pressing and rolling away mid and lower back stiffness we free up the functioning of deep nerve centers (plexus) in the abdomen and pelvis (see the article 47 Messengers). Be alert for sensations of stiffness and vertebrae that may be out of place. Work into and through these feelings; they are your guide.

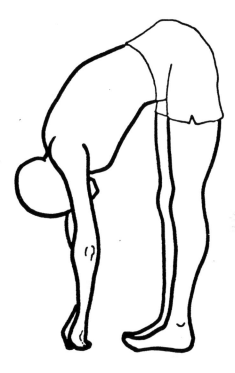

The forward bend uses the body's own weight to stretch the back of the legs, the hips and lower back. Bend forward and let the head and arms fall freely. Keep the legs straight or slightly bent. Let gravity do the work in this stretch and within a minute or so the muscles involved will give and lengthen.

When coming out of this position bend the knees and slowly unwind the body up bit by bit, the head straightening up last. Sense the flexibility and flow in the back as it uncurls into an erect position.

A FINAL NOTE

In some systems of physical liberation the pelvis and abdomen are considered the most difficult parts of the body to release from tension and stiffness. The muscles are so powerful and the feelings contained so strong that for most people it may be just "too hot to handle".

Possibly, before the lower energy centers within the pelvis and belly are opened up, the legs will have to relax some and so will the face and upper body. The process of learning to relax is circular in that our effort and concentration moves around to different parts of the body over the course of time. The lower centers may not be our first object of attention. We may feel the need to release some other tension first.

Inevitably contact will be made with the deeper centers as the body learns to stretch and relax.

Learning to relax is a natural process. It has more to do with an attitude of surrendering to the body than conquering it. The body is not a piece of senseless matter that needs shaping and conditioning. The feelings sensed within our own muscles and joints are ultimately the wisdom and guidance that show us how to live, move, and relax.

BIBLIOGRAPHY

1. HARA, THE VITAL CENTRE OF MAN, Karlfried Durkheim, Samuel Weiser Inc., first English publication 1962.
2. IBID.
3. IBID.
4. EMBRACE TIGER RETURN TO MOUNTAIN, Al Huang, Real People Press, 1973.
5. AIKIDO IN DAILY LIFE, Koichi Tohei, Rikugei Publishing House, 1966.

REFERENCES

ROLFING, THE INTEGRATION OF HUMAN STRUCTURES, Ida P. Rolf, Dennis-Landman publishers, 1977.

ORTHOTHERAPY, Arthur A. Michele, M.D., M. Evans and Company, Inc., 1971.

BODYMIND, Ken Dychtwald, Pantheon, 1977.

THE BODY HAS ITS REASONS, Therese Bertherat and Carol Bernstein, Pantheon, 1977.

DO-IT-YOURSELF SHIATSU (section on Ampuku Therapy), Wataru Ohashi, E.P. Dutton and Co., 1976.

THE BODY REVEALS, Ron Kurtz and Hector Prestera, M.D., Bantam Books, 1977.

THE SECRET OF THE GOLDEN FLOWER, (especially section: The Book of Consciousness and Life), Translated by Richard Wilhelm, Harvest Book, 1962.

OPEN HEART

*Techniques
For Opening
The Heart
Center*

Illustrated
by
Kent Collins
and
Amy Marx

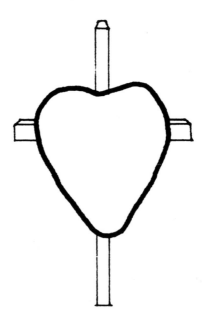

"The little space within the heart is as great as this vast universe. The heavens and earth are there, and the sun, and the moon, and the stars; fire and lightning and winds are there; and all that now is and all that is not: for the whole universe is in Him and He dwells within our heart."

from the Chandogya Upanishad

Someone went up to a madman who was weeping in the bitterest possible way.
He said:
'Why do you cry?'
The madman answered:
'I am crying to attract the pity of His heart.'
The other told him:
'Your words are nonsense, for He has no physical heart.'
The madman answered:
'It is you who are wrong, for He is the owner of all the hearts which exist. Through the heart you can make your connection with God.'

a Sufi story

MIND IN SERVICE TO THE HEART

The English language is full of expressions about the heart. To have heart implies feelings of sympathy and caring. A person with a big heart is loving and generous. To be all heart is to be full of good feeling. From the bottom of the heart means with a great depth of feeling. Frustrated lovers suffer from heartache and to have no heart makes one cruel and heartless. The list can go on.

Many of us think that these are only figures of speech that have nothing much to do with the actual anatomical heart that lies within our chest and pumps blood through our bodies. Yet language often does express with figures of speech an awareness and appreciation of things we may have lost in ourselves or have long forgotten.

The heart is a center for human feelings and emotions. It is not the sum total of being human, just as intellect is not complete in itself, but it is a center that commands and directs much of our energies and focuses and gives direction to our minds.

Strip away the conceptual cover on our emotions and feelings and the heart appears. This is the heart of flesh and blood that beats in our chest. As our awareness deepens and develops we realize it is a heart in much pain. We can sense how uneasy it is.

HEART CENTER

What does feeling this elemental heart soreness mean? It means we have come to the center of emotional diseases and many of our physical ones. We are at the center of our affection for other human beings and our hate for them.

We have found the center of compassion and cruelty. There is the potential for evil in this broken and injured heart but the possibility of freedom and openness exists here too. We have found the center to our emotional storms and the possibility of some peace from them.

THE CROSS AS A HEART SYMBOL

The Christian Cross is a symbol full of power and mystery. By itself or holding the body of Christ, the Cross has drawn or else repelled millions of people for almost two thousand years. It stands as the central symbol of Christianity.

In a very fundamental way the Cross symbolizes Christ's love and suffering and also our own. It has the power to tap into some of our deepest feelings of man's suffering and draw us towards the promise of God's love and forgiveness.

The Cross is a symbol for man. The fact that Christ is often shown nailed to the Cross reinforces this association of the Cross and a man's body. As a symbol of the figure of a man the Cross centers at the heart. The Cross is both a symbol of man and man's heart. Much of Christianity's power and endurance must come from this simple symbol's ability to evoke these strong associations and feelings.

Historically this association becomes conscious in the middle ages when references begin to appear about the Sacred Heart of Jesus. The Sacred Heart of Jesus represents Jesus's love and suffering. It is portrayed as a heart wearing the crown of thorns. Christ's love and particularly his suffering is centered at the heart, his Sacred Heart.

By inference the power of such imagery suggests that all

men and women are wearing a crown of thorns around their hearts. Our personal sense of this may be quite unconscious but the potential to feel this pain is there always. Our heartache makes us seek love and acceptance and yet we never find enough. It makes us cruel and intolerant, desiring hurt and pain for others.

Christianity is a religion of the heart. The issues of Christianity are the heart-centered ones of love and its loss. The image of Christ, nailed to the cross, touches us and our own suffering. It reminds us of our own Sacred Heart of pain.

BELLY CENTER

The heart is not the only center in the body. Almost any organ or point on the body can act as a central focus to consciousness. Yet over the centuries men and women who have explored themselves with concentration and meditation have emphasized certain areas much more than others. The area between the eyes is one such point and it is called the third eye. An inch or two below the navel and slightly inside the abdomen is the "sea of energy" in the Chinese understanding of the body. Where the heart has always been considered the essential center for man in the West, this point below the navel has taken precedence for the far Easterners. Its importance is stressed in their martial practices, their body meditations and their healing arts.

The belly center is our sexual center, a center of healing energy, and the source of the life force in our bodies. It may become conscious to us only after some heart awareness develops or it may precede an awareness of the heart. No hard rules apply in this work. Individual differences will make for very different styles of personal development.

TECHNIQUES FOR OPENING THE HEART CENTER

For thousands of years the Chinese have recognized that internal organs project on the surface of the body. Pain and tenderness at the surface usually reflect a disturbance of an organ inside. To influence the course of disease Eastern medicine will manipulate these areas on the surface by either finger pressure, the heat from burning herbs (moxibustion) or the insertion of needles.

Every major organ has its own special projection. This kind of understanding of the body and its organs develops out of a keen awareness of the kinesthetic or inner body sense. Eastern ways of health and exercise, like yoga or t'ai chi, were developed out of this internal sense. The techniques described here are meant to reawaken the kinesthetic sense and to use it as a guide for opening the heart.

The heart projects on the front of the chest along the sternum. It also projects strongly between the shoulder blades on the back, especially around the first six thoracic vertebrae. Not only will the muscles on either side of the spine be tender and sore here but the vertebrae will frequently misalign in response to disturbances of the heart.

Working the heart begins with manipulation of:
1/the sternum and its periphery
2/the points of tenderness in the musculature of the back between the shoulder blades
3/the first six or seven thoracic vertebrae and also the cervical vertebrae

This work is not always easy or pleasant and is certainly not for everyone. A background in yoga and the meditative arts may be a necessary prerequisite to tolerating and appreciating the sensations. Remember that the discomfort and soreness experienced in these specific points at the body's surface are reflections from the heart itself. This becomes evident in the course of the work. The external tenderness will gradually disappear and a greater sense of the internal heart soreness appears.

Our diseased hearts are not merely the product of our own life histories but in a sense the history of civilized man. When we realize that our twisted and disturbed hearts have been thousands of years in the making, we find the patience for this work. A week, a month or even a year is not a long time considering the centuries it took to create the kind of people we are.

INTERNAL TECHNIQUES

The techniques for opening the heart are not exercises. Exercise works the muscles by rapid and repetitive movements, and it is performed in a spirit of mind dominating and controlling the body. We do push-ups and sit-ups because we were told they were good for us and the more we can do of them the better off we think we are. Exercise is usually a grim and mechanical way to use the body. Internal techniques come from inner (kinesthetic) sensation. They are done in a spirit of relaxation and gentleness, and they allow the body to express its own wants and needs. Internal techniques are closer to physical therapy than to exercise. The sense of stiffness and tension acts as a guide; the body is treated gently and with respect. Instead of using force, the body is coaxed and eased into stretching and moving. Animals and young children move this way. Their egos are rudimentary or nonexistent and they haven't lost touch with the wisdom of their kinesthetic sense.

TOOLS

Two basic tools are used for opening the heart associated areas on the body. The basic spinal roller is any large and firm roller. A spinal roller can be constructed by using a large rolling pin tightly rolled into one or two regular towels folded in half. The cushioning is important to prevent bruising and injury but the quality of firmness given by the hard rolling pin inside is necessary to accomplish the task of manipulating the chest and back. Once the roller is made it should be secured with two or three strong elastics to keep the towels in place.

The other tools are any hard rubber balls from 1½" to 2½" in diameter. These balls should be very firm with very little squish or give to them. Handballs (specifically for the game of handball, not raquetballs or paddleballs) or lacrosse balls are the most ideal ones commercially available. Some toy rubber balls will also work adequately as long as they are about 2" in diameter and quite solid. These balls will be used to press into the heart-associated points on either side of the spine on the back.

ROLLING THE CHEST

Supporting yourself on your hands and knees press the roller into the middle of your chest on the sternum. Gradually and gently roll up and down on your sternum. The weight of your body gives sufficient force to the manipulation and one should use the strength in the arms to adjust the amount of body weight applied to the chest. Be cautious but be aware of what you feel.

There may be pain and discomfort at points along the sternum. Do not go beyond your tolerable threshold of pain but do feel the aches and stiffness that probably reside there in your chest. Press and roll over those sore areas. Work only a minute or two at first. After two or three weeks your arms will get stronger and your skill and awareness in this internal technique will increase. It may take weeks or months to release and loosen the stiffness found here. Be patient but persistent.

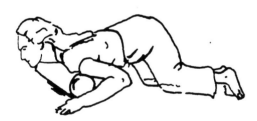

MASSAGING THE CHEST

Rolling the chest may awaken you to points and areas of soreness along, around and on top of the sternum. By using one or both hands in the traditional prayer position (with the bony protrusion at the very base of the thumb against the chest) these points can be firmly pressed and massaged.

Explore along the sides of the sternum and on the sternum itself. Try to locate those points of tenderness brought out into awareness by the roller. Press these points strongly and massage them with small circular motions. Search out other tender spots along the base of the clavicle and between the ribs. These, too, can be pressed and massaged.

While we are discovering our pain and tension, we are also treating it. Eventually all pain and points of soreness should disappear although it may take some time. Remember to be gentle and patient with yourself.

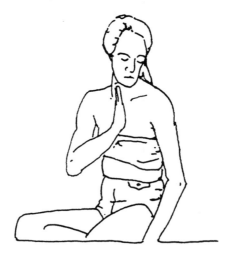

PRESSING THE HEART POINTS ON THE BACK

Place two hard rubber balls on a firm floor. Too much cushioning or a thick carpet may absorb the balls and take away from the pressure applied to the back. Put the balls on either side of the spine at the top of the shoulders. Arch up on the two balls. Roll the balls down an inch or so at a time and press them into the muscles running along either side of the spine. For some people using one ball at a time may be easier.

A great deal of tension and stiffness has settled in between the shoulder blades of many of us. These muscles have become hard and tough and literally full of pain and sensitivity when sufficiently manipulated. All this pain and sensitivity is often a reflection from the heart and lungs. The hardness, resistance and discomfort found between the shoulder blades can be worked out but it usually takes a couple of months of steady work.

We have come a long way from being in a state of natural health and ease; it takes time and persistence to make our way back.

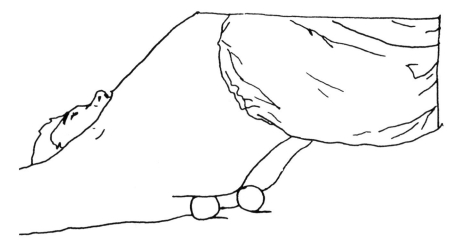

MANIPULATING THE SPINE

The spine will twist and distort in response to back and chest tension and to soreness in the heart. A complete therapeutic approach will have to include work on the spine. It is very possible to relieve spinal distortion and stiffness by spinal rolling and self-manipulation techniques.

A firm slightly cushioned floor offers an excellent opportunity for rolling and massaging the back. Feel for areas of pain and stiffness and where vertebrae may seem out of place. Roll over and press into these areas. The back may even snap and crunch as vertebrae are pushed back into alignment. The sense of ache and stiffness will also be relieved as one rolls on and presses into the back.

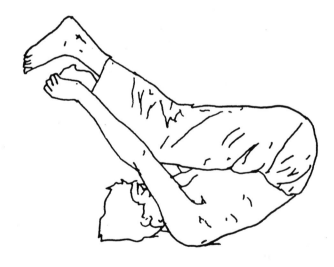

A spinal roller adds a sharper dimension to spinal rolling. Put the roller at the top of the shoulders and arch up onto it. Roll the roller an inch or two at a time down the entire back. Again feel for the areas of stiffness, pain and resistance. The roller can focus pressure directly between the vertebrae. The first five or six thoracic vertebrae relate to the heart and lungs. Aches and stiffness here reflect the condition of the heart and lungs and also can affect their condition.

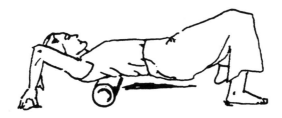

The neck also contains important nerve centers (the cervical ganglia and the cardiac nerves, see the article 47 Messengers) that stress the heart. Be sure to press the roller between the cervical vertebrae to loosen, relax and adjust the neck.

Go slowly and cautiously at first until one is familiar and comfortable with these sensations and the techniques. The stress and distortion in our chest, shoulders, neck and back can be tremendous. Gradually and gently probe the depths of pain and distortion here. Allow these feelings to emerge into the light of consciousness but do it slowly and with care.

MANIPULATION FOR THE SHOULDERS AND ARMS

Besides projecting on the back and chest the heart projects into the shoulders and down the arms. Anyone who has ever suffered severe angina or even a heart attack is made aware of the extent of the heart's influence and projection. As our awareness of the heart center increases we will naturally be more inclined to stretch the arms, shoulders and chest.

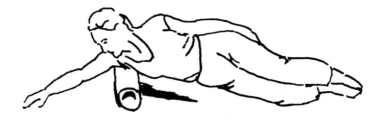

The roller can be used to press into the shoulder joint and to massage the surrounding muscles.

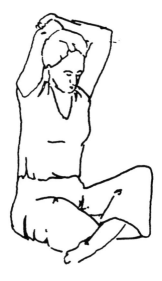

Pull the elbow across the back of the head to stretch the arm and shoulder.

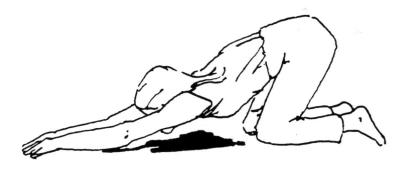

This deep bowing position stretches the chest muscles and the arms.

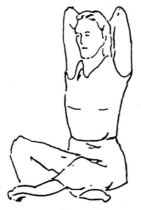

Here both elbows are brought up over the head and stretched backwards. The back of the arms are given a good stretch and the chest is opened.

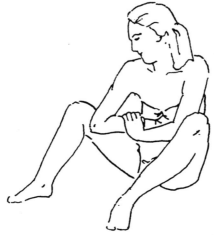

The back of the wrist is against the side of the waist. The elbow is placed inside the thigh. The other hand presses the forearm gently down against the thigh. This is a strong stretch and manipulation for the shoulder joint and the surrounding muscles, tendons and ligaments.

THE HAND

The hand contains specific areas that reflect the condition of the internal organs and other parts of the body. If the other heart related points are indeed tender and sore then there is a good chance that the heart related area on the hand will also be sore.

Press this spot on the hand strongly with the tip of your thumb or else press a small, hard rubber ball into the spot. It may well be extremely tender. With time and patient manipulation this point of pain on the hand will eventually disappear.

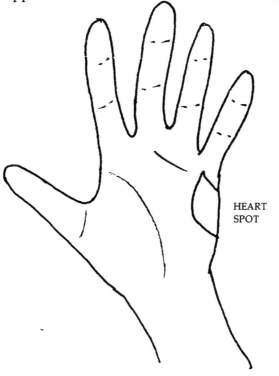

HEART
SPOT

THE HEART IN MEDITATION

By themselves these techniques will not open the heart. They will awaken us to the heart's condition and eventually alleviate the external soreness associated with the heart's discomfort. As the tensions and physical distortions are relieved, the internal body sense moves into the heart itself.

Techniques and manipulation can take us just so far. They are tools for growth but at times they must be abandoned as we learn to surrender and let go. Our struggle to free our hearts is also part of the problem. The struggle must end. We are left with our essential heartache and no power to affect it except by our own awareness.

In moments of stillness, rest and meditation we are drawn into this painful core. Consciousness fills with this hurt inside our chest. We have encountered an elemental level of human affliction in ourselves and have embarked on the cure.

REFERENCES

BOOK OF SECRETS BOOK I, Bhagwan Shree Rajneesh, Harper and Row, 1974.

AWAKEN HEALING ENERGY THROUGH THE TAO, Mantak Chia, Copen Press, 1981.

HARA, THE VITAL CENTRE OF MAN, Karlfried Durkheim, Samuel Weiser Inc., 1962.

DO-IT-YOURSELF SHIATSU, Wataru Ohashi, Dutton, 1976.

ZEN SHIATSU, Shizuto Masunaga, Japan Publications, Inc., 1977.

ACUPUNCTURE, Felix Mann, Vintage, 1962.

BASIC STRUCTURAL YOGA, Tom Stiles, Collected Consciousness, 1975.

THE MEANING OF CHRIST, Robert Clyde Johnson, Westminster Press, 1968.

THE UPANISHADS, translation by Juan Mascaro, Penguin, 1965.

THE WAY OF THE SUFI, Idries Shah, Octagon Press, 1968.

BREATH, SLEEP, THE HEART AND LIFE, Pundit Acharya, Dawn Horse Press, 1975.

When all desires that cling to the heart are surrendered, then a mortal becomes immortal, and even in this world he is one with Brahman.

When all the ties that bind the heart are unloosened, then a mortal becomes immortal. This is the sacred teaching.

One hundred and one subtle ways come from the heart. One of them rises to the crown of the head. This is the way that leads to immortality; the others lead to different ends.

Always dwelling within all beings is the Atman, the Purusha, the Self, a little flame in the heart. Let one with steadiness withdraw him from the body even as an inner stem is withdrawn from its sheath. Know this pure immortal light; know in truth this pure immortal light.

from the Katha Upanishad

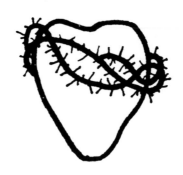

DOOR
OF
LIFE

*Lumbar Spine
Stretch And
Manipulation*

DOOR OF LIFE

In Chinese yoga and meditation the middle of the lumbar spine between the second and third lumbar vertebrae is an area called the Door of Life. This point between the vertebrae is considered the principle power point of the body and traditionally it has been associated with the kidneys. Pressure and manipulation to this location on the spine and other spots in the general vicinity is the recommended treatment for revitalizing the entire body. More than any other point on the body, pressure on this area in the lower back increases the charge of life energy that expresses itself in movement, sexuality and healing.

OPENING THE DOOR

This charge of life energy is usually experienced as sexual excitement yet can also be felt as the life force in our bodies. As physical awareness deepens, this center in the pit of our abdomen is sensed as the energy center of the body. Sexuality is the nearest and easiest expression of this energy but not the only possibility for it. This energy or charge can move and expand and in Chinese healing practices it can circulate thru the spine, head, chest and limbs. This is an energy that circulates in our body and on which so much of our health and well-being depends. Block this energy or let it stagnate and ill-health will soon follow.

Most people block their basic life energy. Western psychology has expressed it in terms of the repression of libido. This repression, as the word aptly suggests, is a clamp or a pressure applied upon the charge of feeling and energy in the depths of our abdomen. We learn to control ourselves at five or six years of age by containing the flow of energy and impulse that begins in our belly. We do this to please our parents and to eventually fit into the culture. The demands of our society are such that a great deal of control and containment are necessary to function and to relate to others.

We sacrifice the fullness of our physical power to fit into society. We are all suffering from a diminished capacity to feel and to be our natural selves. This diminished capacity can be experienced as pain and tension, and the pain and stiffness that so many people feel in their low backs is part of a pattern of tension that presses down on a sea of energy in our abdomen.

This pattern of tension is particularly strong in the lower back, abdomen and the inside of the thighs. It is an attempt to cap a fountain of charged energy flow with tension and internal pressure. To one extent or another all civilized people suffer from this maneuver, this squeezing of life.

The most effective way to diminish our life's energy is to tense the back. Tensing the back is a natural reaction to stress, but maintain that tension and eventually the spine itself will compress and distort. This distortion in the spine is also part of the clamp restricting the flow of our life energy. Open and lengthen the spine, particularly in the lumbar area, and the fountain of energy in our depths will be released. This is the inner meaning to calling the center of our lumbar spine the Door of Life.

This is not a quick and easy task. We have much of our social and personal identity invested in our tension and, in a sense, stretching the spine and back muscles is going against the current of our education and training. The extreme stiffness in our backs represents our accumulated socialization and repression. The process of opening and letting go is often part of maturity and adulthood. It can be our principle preoccupation in later life as we increasingly "see through" our conditioning and training to something more essential underneath.

KNEES TO CHEST AND HOLD

The first and most basic stretch available to us for our low back is knees-to-chest and hold. If you like, put a pillow underneath the head to prevent the neck from shortening and tightening as it might in this position. The knees are drawn up as far as is comfortable and held for 30 seconds or a minute. The steady but gentle holding of the position is what creates the stretch and lengthening of the lumbar area. Stretching too rapidly with bouncing or forcefully applied bursts of movement will not lengthen the spine and muscles, but will likely tighten them more.

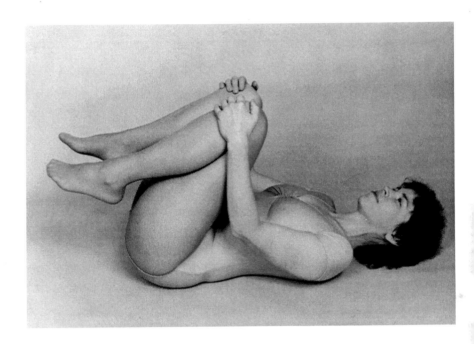

This position delivers a traction effect to the lower back. For a longer stretch the knees can be secured in position by an overlarge belt or a large strip of cloth drawn around the middle of the back and tied over the knees. The arms then can relax down by the sides of the body.

If there is spinal distortion, the hips and legs will tilt to one side or another. Make slight rocking motions from side to side and this will massage and adjust the low back against the surface underneath.

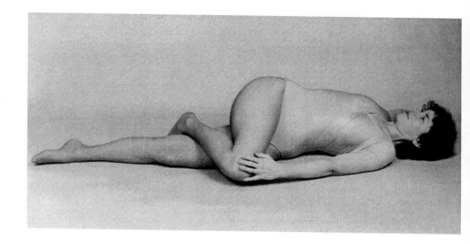

SPINAL TWIST

Put the instep of one foot against the back of the other knee. Draw the bent knee down towards the floor as far as is comfortable. Allow the free arm to fall back diagonally away from the body. This is the classic chiropractic position used for lumbar adjustment; you may feel this adjustment as you practice this position.

Again hold the position for 30 seconds. Feel the stretch in your chest muscles as the free arm stretches up and back. Wiggle your hips back and forth slightly to increase the loosening action in the back and hips.

THE SPINAL ROLLER

The spinal roller is any large, firm roller with sufficient cushioning to prevent bruising and injury. A homemade roller can be constructed by wrapping two folded towels tightly around a good size rolling pin. The firmness of the device is important because too soft a roller will not apply the direct pressure to the points between the vertebrae that is necessary for this kind of treatment.

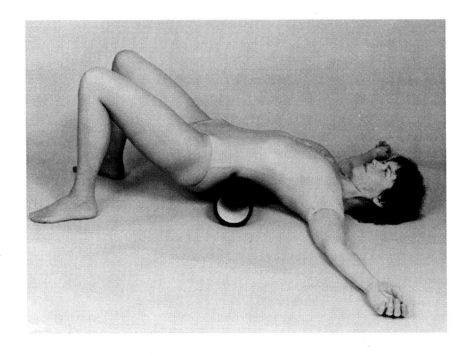

In the photograph a roller is being used to press and gently roll the lumbar spine and the lower thoracic spine. Be alert to sensations of stiffness and vertebrae out of place. These sensations indicate blockage and the need for pressure and manipulation.

Between the 11th thoracic and the 3rd lumbar vertebrae the kidneys and the adrenal glands are found. Stiffness here can lead to a host of physical problems from high blood pressure to allergies. Be gentle with yourself in this work and do not expect to relieve misalignments and tension in a day or even a week. Be patient with yourself; be gentle.

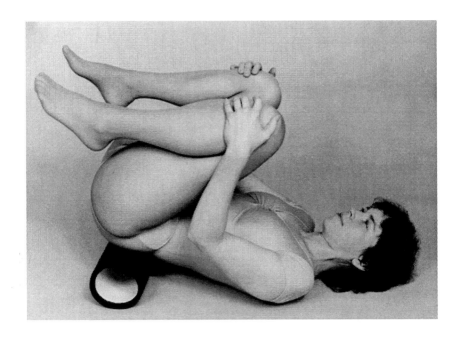

KNEES TO CHEST WITH ROLLER

With the roller underneath the hips, pull the knees to your chest. This is the same position as knees to chest and hold, but with the roller underneath the hips the traction effect for the lower back is increased.

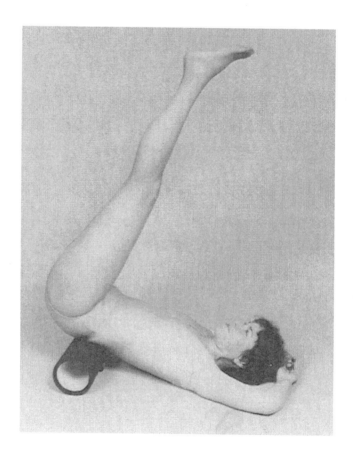

SHOULDER STAND WITH ROLLER

As your flexibility increases try doing a shoulder stand with the roller placed at about the 11th or 12th thoracic vertebrae. This is about where the adrenal glands are found. Hold the position and allow the roller to press between the vertebrae. Now move the roller down an inch at a time and let it press into the lumbar spine and into the sacrum. Be alert to any sensations of pain and discomfort. Pain alerts us to blockage and distortion.

Remember that between the 2nd and 3rd lumbar vertebrae is a spot called the Door of Life. You are knocking on this door and with patience and gentle persistence it will open.

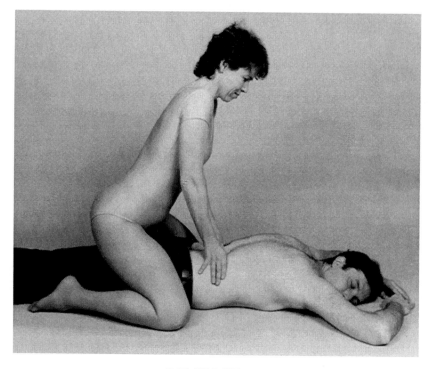

MASSAGE

Strong direct pressure with the heel of the hands or with the thumbs against the muscles of the back can be an effective therapy. This kind of pressure is best applied with the recipient on the floor. The therapist leans her weight into the recipient. Her arms remain relatively straight.

The thumbs are being pressed into the muscles along the lumbar spine. Most back pain is due to muscle spasm and tightness; explore along the muscles that lie next to the spine for hard, stiff areas that are also sensitive to pressure. Press these points of sensitivity and massage them. Massage on these pressure points will induce muscle tension and stiffness to release.

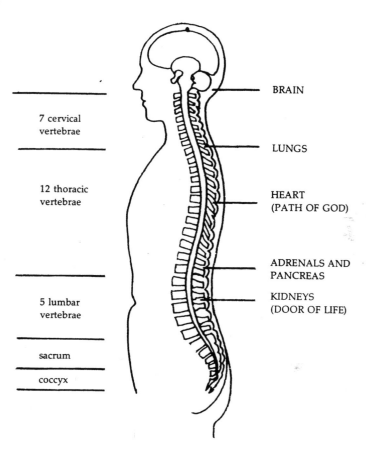

7 cervical vertebrae

12 thoracic vertebrae

5 lumbar vertebrae

sacrum

coccyx

BRAIN

LUNGS

HEART
(PATH OF GOD)

ADRENALS AND PANCREAS

KIDNEYS
(DOOR OF LIFE)

CENTERS IN THE SPINE

This is a chart of some of the well recognized centers in the spine according to Oriental medicine. The organs related to these centers are shown. Note that the heart center is also referred to as Path of God and the kidney center as Door of Life, suggesting the importance of these points in one's growth and development. These centers in the spine can become blocked affecting the internal organ function and general well-being.

REFERENCES

BOOK OF SECRETS BOOK I, Bhagwan Shree Rajneesh, Harper and Row, 1974.

AWAKEN HEALING ENERGY THROUGH THE TAO, Mantak Chia, Copen Press, 1981.

HARA, THE VITAL CENTRE OF MAN, Karlfried Durkheim, Samuel Weiser Inc., 1962.

DO-IT-YOURSELF SHIATSU, Wataru Ohashi, Dutton, 1976.

TSUBO, VITAL POINTS FOR ORIENTAL THERAPY, Katsusuke Serizawa, Japan Publications Inc., 1976.

DISTORTION
AND
ADJU<u>S</u>TMENT

Ten
Principles

BEING BROKEN

Training a horse to take a rider on its back is called breaking the horse. In human beings a similar process occurs when the young child is taught to inhibit impulses and feelings. The great energy and movement in young children must be channeled into socially acceptable paths. This process of channeling impulse and energy can at times be so severe that the child actually incurs an internal injury trying to meet the demands placed on him by parents and society.

For many of us this injury and the decreased vitality it creates is a foundation to the kind of individual who can fit into society and who can identify with the things the society offers.

TENSION AND DISTORTION

Almost any adult body upon close inspection will exhibit areas of tension and distortion. Spines appear crooked; heads seem to be falling forward. Specific vertebrae noticeably jut out from the smooth curves of the back. The chest is crushed or permanently blown up; ribs and sternum stick out or sink in. The round, smooth and even contours that usually spell health are not to be found but instead are replaced by constriction and jagged edges.

Moderate pressure almost anywhere elicits pain. Pain will be found at the base of the skull, in the muscles along either side of the spine and between the vertebrae. The hands and feet are filled with sensitivity, the connections between the sternum and ribs are sore, the abdomen is hard, lumpy and tender. Even the top of the head can be painful to the touch. The all too frequent human condition is full of tension, distortion and pain.

DIVERTED ATTENTION

The demands of education, work and social responsibility divert our attention away from an awareness of this condition of tension and distortion. The large cerebral cortex in man looks out onto the world and tries to understand and to change it. Technological civilization has changed the face of the earth to suit human needs and desire and yet the cost of this achievement is a kind of blindness to our essential nature. This blindness can be fatal. For the individual it leads to neurosis and disease. For a society it leads to increasing social discord, general perversity and aggression and eventually to its own destruction.

REDIRECTING ATTENTION
THE SEVENTH SENSE

By quieting cerebral activity and learning to focus awareness towards an internal environment the extent of our tension and distortion can be felt. Our seventh sense (after seeing, hearing, smelling, tasting, touching and balancing) is called the kinesthetic sense. If the dominance of the other senses can be toned down, the kinesthetic sense can appear. The kinesthetic sense is an awareness of the tension in our muscles and the stiffness in our joints. It shows us where the flow of energy and feeling is blocked and how and where we are harboring disease.

Being in touch with our kinesthetic sense means having depth and possessing the key to growth and change.

THE SPONTANEOUS HEALING PROCESS

With this key, this kinesthetic awareness of our internal environment, we tap into the wisdom and guidance inside our bodies. We come to know what it means to be spontaneous and natural as our actions and feelings increasingly come from our depths. Life then proceeds, at its own pace, on an evolutionary journey towards liberation.

Like peeling off the layers of an onion, our tension and distortion is removed in stages. This is not a process that requires the use of force or the application of willpower but only the allowance of and surrender to an unfolding, a de-kinking, a softening and relaxing. The body has always wanted to indulge itself in this healing process but we may never have let it. Now with our internal focus sharpened, this indulgence seems the only course of action that makes any sense.

PAIN AS A GUIDE

What punctuates and guides our healing process is pain. This is a pain that attacks us in many places and with differing intensity. We may have vaguely sensed a discomfort and uneasiness before, but as our ability to indulge in a spontaneous healing process grows we sense the full extent of our suffering and pain.

Like an injured animal we instinctively respond to this pain. We stretch and roll; we cry and moan and sigh. We press on spots that feel sore.

Our sheer exhaustion may emerge and like cats we languish and repose for twenty hours a day. For all the world this is a waste of time and a case of laziness but we move to a different drummer.

BREAKING UP STIFFNESS AND TENSION

The more active and purposeful part of our healing process is really a measured and gently applied program of self-destruction. None of us know how to fix ourselves exactly, but with a sharper insight into specific areas of tension and stiffness we can focus an attack. This is an attack designed to gradually destroy the body that we have known. We tear it down, rip it up and start over again. By destroying the structure and character of our distorted bodies we allow ourselves to take on a new shape.

What this new shape will be we cannot precisely know. During periods of sleep and rest (those times for repair and renewal) we will slowly progress towards a new openness and freedom. Each tension untied and stiffness loosened becomes a step towards new health and increased vitality.

FREEING ORGANS

As awareness, our kinesthetic sense, matures and deepens, we may discover an aspect of our true nature that Chinese medicine has recognized for at least two thousand years: that life in the body is an expression of internal organs and that health and vitality are built on the free functioning of those organs. Our organs are filled with power and it is up to us to release this power for the sake of our own well-being. This power in organs is our birthright and though we may have had this power once, when young, it is soon driven out of our system.

Chinese medicine sees the condition at the surface of the body as a reflection of internal function. Internal organs have an influence and effect down into the hands and feet, and so the tenderness we find in the hands and feet often refer to disturbances in internal function. Points along either side of the spine can be very tender; these points are called associated points because they are intimately associated with internal organ function. What may at first seem to be merely a loosening of an area of pain and stiffness is in fact an organ expressing its desire to be free. This becomes increasingly evident as we allow the process to unfold. Lungs, heart, glands, digestion, nerves and brain come alive; each contributing tremendous power to the new and revitalized creature emerging.

USING TOOLS

One can imagine the evolution of the development of acupuncture. Long before sharp and penetrating needles were inserted into specific points, people were using their fingers and nails to press spots that were sore or felt tense. Acupuncture must certainly have evolved out of a system of massage and manipulation. Even today professional acupuncturists will manipulate with their fingers first to locate those tender and sensitive spots that indicate blockage and disturbance. These are the points most often needled.

As ancient therapists became more familiar with the map of possible points, they began to experiment with different devices that could even more effectively free the snagged and thwarted spots to be found in the body. No doubt sticks and stones, sharp ones and blunt ones, were used. The ancient manipulators probably gathered together quite a collection of tools, each particularly effective for a certain area.

With tools greater force, leverage and focus can be applied to the problem of tension and distortion. With the application of ever sharper therapeutic tools the science of massage and manipulation evolves, the most refined and subtle development being acupuncture itself.

THE TOOL KIT

Rediscovering those roots to Chinese therapy is an adventure in personal development. Like the ancients we, too, can discover how the leverage and focus that tools provide can greatly enhance our quest for physical and mental liberation. Man is unique among animals by his extensive use of tools, and it is the unique man and woman who can effectively use tools on his or her own body. Using tools brings our suffering (tension, stiffness and distortion) into focus and certainly must accelerate our evolution towards health and happiness.

The tool kit shown on this page includes: a rubber-cushioned Spinal Roller for manipulation of the spine; a Ma Roller for the organ associated points along either side of the spine; two sizes of hard rubber balls for these same points; a ridged foot roller; a Cranial Adjustor and Cervical Wedge for the head, base of the skull and cervical region; and three wooden dowels with rounded ends for applying pressure, rolling and striking movements.

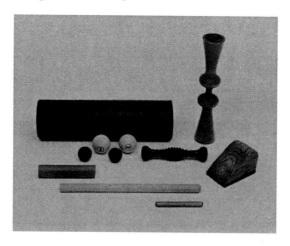

REFERENCES

AQUARIAN AGE HEALING, Hurley and Sanders, Health Research, 1963.

BIOENGINEERING, Hurley and Sanders, Health Research, 1970.

ROLFING, THE INTEGRATION OF HUMAN STRUCTURES, Ida P. Rolf, Dennis-Landman Publishers, 1977.

THE BODY REVEALS, Ron Kurtz and Hector Prestera, M.D., Bantam Books, 1977.

MAN IN THE TRAP, Elsworth F. Baker, M.D., Avon Books, 1967.

AWAKEN HEALING ENERGY THROUGH THE TAO, Mantak Chia, Copen Press, 1981.

THE BOOK OF DO-IN, Michio Kushi, Japan Publications, 1979.

DO-IT-YOURSELF SHIATSU, Wataru Ohashi, E.P. Dutton and Co., 1976.

BASIC STRUCTURAL YOGA, Tom Stiles, Collected Consciousness, 1976.

BRILLIANT FUNCTION OF PAIN, Milton Ward, Optimus Books, 1977.

THE HISTORICAL DEVELOPMENT OF ACUPUNCTURE, Chuang Yu-Min, Oriental Healing Arts Institute, 1982.

RESTORE VITALITY THRU ADRENAL MASSAGE

More than any other organ in the body the adrenal glands prepare the body to meet the demands of life. Scientific research over the last fifty years has shown that prolonged stress has a dramatic effect on the adrenal glands. Under prolonged stress the adrenals noticeably swell to meet the increased demand for their energy-giving, life-sustaining hormones.

The inner part of the adrenals, called the adrenal medulla, produces adrenalin and noradrenalin. These powerful hormones stimulate and mobilize the body for action. These hormones increase the power of the heart and open and relax the lungs. Medically adrenalin is frequently used in cases of shock and in severe asthmatic conditions.

The adrenal cortex or outer part of the gland produces a large variety of hormones, six or seven of which are particularly important and active. The anti-inflammatory (glucocorticoids) are especially important in the general adaption of the body to stress. These hormones, besides increasing blood sugar levels, inhibit the formation of inflammatory conditions.

Although our bodies can adapt to long term stress, our capacity to stand up to prolonged stress is finite. At some point our resistance, which may last for months or years, will break down. This breakdown is characterized by a breakdown and exhaustion of adrenal function. No longer able to respond to life's demands, the complex battery of hormones that sustain our vitality and give balance to our lives fail to do their job properly and we become ill. Respiration becomes more difficult, the heart lacks power. We become susceptible to inflammatory conditions that may arise almost anywhere in the body. Life loses its resiliency and power.

Three measures can be taken to help restore the adrenal glands to normal function. First, sufficient rest is necessary. Much of human stress is self-induced and a person needs to recognize if he or she is living too fast and driving too hard. This is the hardest lesson to learn. Slow down, be kind and gentle to yourself, lay down and relax during the day, get sufficient sleep at night. Learn to recognize that the increased pace and intensity of modern life may diminish the natural span of life.

A balanced diet, particularly rich in B vitamins, is important. A poor diet lacking any of the essential nutrients can lead to disease and exhaustion. Pantothenic acid, one of the B vitamins, has been experimentally shown to affect adrenal function.

Lastly, direct manipulation properly applied over the adrenals can powerfully affect their recovery. For severely depleted adrenals diet and rest alone will probably not be enough. Direct stimulation to the correct adrenal points on the back will revive them and go a long way in restoring the body to healthy functioning.

Areas over the adrenals can be quite tender, suggesting the imbalance and disturbance of the glandular structure underneath. Chinese medicine has known for thousands of years how restorative manipulation and pressure over the adrenal glands can be. Not knowing exactly why, but through experimentation, Chinese physicians observed how the whole body could be revitalized by properly applied pressure and manipulation.

Called the Door of Life this area over the kidneys was believed to be the source of our essence and vitality. Western medical research may be coming to the same conclusion. The adrenals increasingly appear to be the axis around which our response to stress revolves.

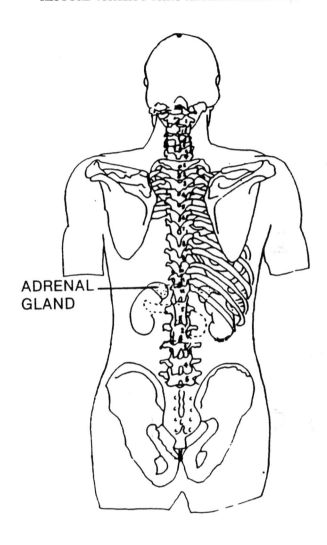

ADRENAL
GLAND

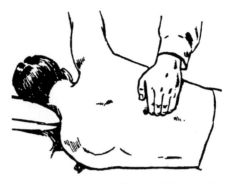

A competent chiropractor or physical therapist should be able to perform adrenal manipulations. Here the patient is lying on his side while the therapist presses firmly into the adrenal area with his fingertips.

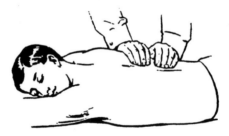

The patient is lying on his stomach while the therapist presses and massages over the kidney and adrenal area. The adrenals usually can be found just underneath the bottom of the rib cage of the back.

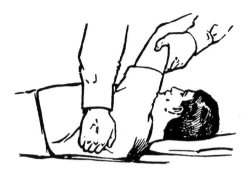

The patient is lying on his back while the therapist presses his fingertips up against the adrenals. Anyone with sufficient strength and flexibility can himself reach around in this position and massage the adrenals with the knuckles of his fist. Search for tender spots and press them with the knuckles. The object is to eventually dispel all traces of soreness although this may take weeks to accomplish. Be patient with yourself. Massage each adrenal area for only two or three minutes a day for the first few weeks. Notice how after a few treatments one's level of vitality and energy increases.

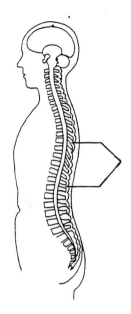

This is the area of the spine that affects adrenal function. The greater, lesser and smallest splanchnic nerves emerge here from the gangliated cord of the sympathetic nervous system. The splanchnic nerves unite to form the solar plexus in the upper abdominal region. It is from the solar plexus, the largest nerve plexus in the body, that the adrenal glands receive their nerve stimulation. (See diagram of the sympathetic nervous system on page 82.)

Stiffness and tension in this area of the back can affect and can also reflect the state of our adrenal glands. Recurrent stiffness here suggests adrenal exhaustion. By loosening and adjusting this section of the back we begin to restore our adrenals to a normal and balanced functioning.

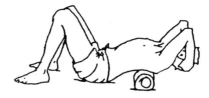

Make a spinal roller by wrapping a small folded towel around a rolling pin. Secure the towel with elastic bands. The roller should be firm enough to apply pressure between the vertebrae. Roll and press the adrenal associated area of the spine between the fifth and twelfth thoracic vertebrae. Feel for specific areas of pain and stiffness. Gradually over weeks and months the stiffness will be rolled away.

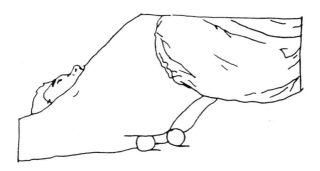

Press two hard rubber balls into the adrenal associated area of the back on either side of the spine. Lacrosse balls are ideal for this kind of self-massage but any comparable hard rubber ball will do. Feel for tension and pain in the muscles alongside the spine. Massage with care and patience these points of tension and they will eventually be massaged away.

REFERENCES

THE STRESS OF LIFE, Hans Selye, M.D., McGraw Hill, 1976.

GRAY'S ANATOMY, Henry Gray, Crown publishers, 1977.

AWAKEN HEALING ENERGY THROUGH THE TAO, Mantak Chia, Copen Press, 1981.

DO-IT-YOURSELF SHIATSU, Wataru Ohashi, Dutton, 1976.

TSUBO, VITAL POINTS FOR ORIENTAL THERAPY, Katsusuke Serizawa, Japan Publications Inc., 1976.

LET'S EAT RIGHT TO KEEP FIT, Adelle Davis, Signet, 1970.

FUNCTIONAL HYPOADRENIA, Dynamic Communications, 1977.

47
MESSENGERS

A Theory On The Origin
And Cure Of Disease

THE SYMPATHETIC SYSTEM OF NERVES

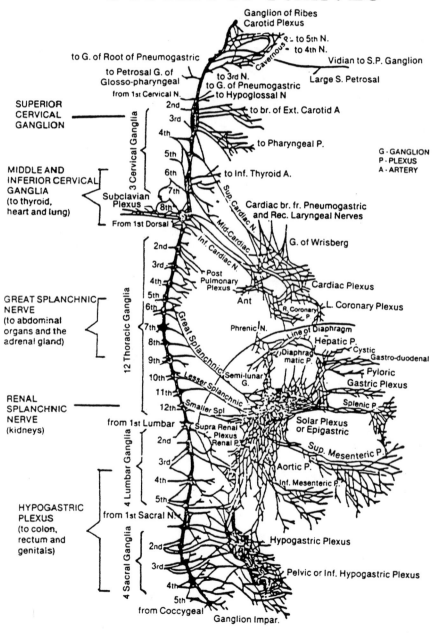

Ganglion of Ribes
Carotid Plexus

P : to 5th N.
to 4th N.

to G. of Root of Pneumogastric
Vidian to S.P. Ganglion

to Petrosal G. of
Glosso-pharyngeal
from 1st Cervical N.

Large S. Petrosal

to 3rd N.
to G. of Pneumogastric
to Hypoglossal N

**SUPERIOR
CERVICAL
GANGLION**

2nd
3rd
4th

to br. of Ext. Carotid A.

to Pharyngeal P.

3 Cervical Ganglia

5th
6th

to Inf. Thyroid A.

G · GANGLION
P · PLEXUS
A · ARTERY

**MIDDLE AND
INFERIOR CERVICAL
GANGLIA
(to thyroid,
heart and lung)**

7th

Subclavian
Plexus

8th

From 1st Dorsal

Sup. Cardiac N.

Mid-Cardiac

Cardiac br. fr. Pneumogastric
and Rec. Laryngeal Nerves

G. of Wrisberg

2nd
3rd
4th
5th
6th
7th
8th
9th
10th
11th
12th

Inf. Cardiac N.

Post
Pulmonary
Plexus

Ant

Cardiac Plexus

R. Coronary
P.

L. Coronary Plexus

**GREAT SPLANCHNIC
NERVE
(to abdominal
organs and the
adrenal gland)**

12 Thoracic Ganglia

Great Splanchnic

Phrenic N.

Line of Diaphragm

Hepatic P.

Cystic

Diaphrag-
matic P.

Gastro-duodenal

Lesser Splanchnic

Semi-lunar
G.

Pyloric

Gastric Plexus

**RENAL
SPLANCHNIC
NERVE
(kidneys)**

Smaller Spl

from 1st Lumbar

Supra Renal
Plexus
Renal P.

Splenic P.

Solar Plexus
or Epigastric

2nd

Sup. Mesenteric P.

4 Lumbar Ganglia

3rd

Aortic P.

4th

Inf. Mesenteric P.

5th

**HYPOGASTRIC
PLEXUS
(to colon,
rectum and
genitals)**

from 1st Sacral N.

4 Sacral Ganglia

2nd

Hypogastric Plexus

3rd

Pelvic or Inf. Hypogastric Plexus

4th
5th

from Coccygeal

Ganglion Impar.

THE SYMPATHETIC NERVOUS SYSTEM

Dr. Richard Selzer in his book *Confessions of a Knife* offers us a description of the Sympathetic nervous system:

"Lying upon the front of each of the vertebrae, from the base of the skull to the tip of the coccyx, is a paired chain of tiny nodes, each of which is connected to the spinal cord and to each other. From these nodes, bundles of nerves extend to meet at relay stations scattered in profusion throughout the body. These ganglia are in anatomical touch with their fellows by a system of circuitry complex and various enough to confound into self-destruction a whole race of computers. Here all is chemical rush and wave-to-wave ripple. Here is fear translated for the flesh, and pride and jealousy. Here dwell zeal and ardor. And love is contracted. By microscopic nervelets, the impulses are carried to all the capillaries, hair follicles and sweat glands of the body. The smooth muscle of the intestine, the lachrymal glands, the bladder and the gentalia are all subject to the bombardment that issues from this vibrating harp of knobs and strings. Innumerable are the orders delivered: Constrict! Dilate! Secrete! Stand erect! It is all very busy, effervescent."

These nodes or ganglia that lie in close to the vertebrae are usually 23 in number on each side of the spine. These two cords of ganglia unite and form a single small ganglia in front of the coccyx. Together they form a system of approximately 47 ganglia; these are the two gangliated cords of the Sympathetic nervous system.

The Sympathetic nervous system is perhaps the most primitive part of our nervous system. Even before animals evolved backbones and spines a system of ganglia and nerves served to order and regulate invertebrate bodies. In the evolution of the nervous system of higher animals these more primitive structures do not disappear. Additional nerve tissue is added on in the form of spines and brains but in all of us this ancient and primitive system of ganglia and nerves continues to exist and to exert its influence.

The Sympathetic nervous system consists then of 47 interconnected ganglia lying close to the vertebrae of our spine. Innumerable nerves branch out from each of the ganglia; some of these branches communicate with the spinal nerves, others communicate with other ganglia and still others penetrate into the depths of the body and form 3 large plexus or aggregates of nerves that regulate internal organ functioning.

THE PARASYMPATHETIC

Our internal organs, including blood vessels, glands, digestive organs, heart and lungs all are largely regulated by either the Sympathetic system or by the other half of our autonomic nervous system, the Parasympathetic. The Parasympathetic consists of 4 pairs of nerves that originate in the medulla and pons of our brains and also nerves originating in the sacral section of our spinal cord. Usually these two components of our autonomic nervous system, the Sympathetic and Parasympathetic, oppose each other in their effects. The Parasympathetic usually controls our functioning during periods of rest and repose. The Parasympathetic slows the heart, increases the action of digestion, and generally allows the body to repair, rest and recuperate.

AN ALARMING MESSAGE

The Sympathetic nervous system, on the other hand, delivers a very different message to the body. This is the message to mobilize and prepare for action. It tells the body that there may be a need to fight or flee and that physical exertion may be necessary. It is a message that tones, excites and braces the body for action. This is the bodily response commonly called stress.

Sympathetic ganglia have connections with the spinal nerves and so affect the voluntary muscles of our body by increasing tension and our ability to quickly respond to demanding situations. When our Sympathetic nerves turn on, the heart is stimulated, breathing quickens, digestion is inhibited and blood pressure rises as blood is directed out of the abdominal viscera into our brains and muscles. Adrenalin is discharged into our blood system reinforcing (by its action on all the cells of the body) the whole complex of responses that go to make up the Sympathetic (stress) response.

SYMPATHETICOTONIA

The Sympathetic response may have been quite appropriate for creatures living in the wild and facing danger or the need to hunt for a living. For modern man this dramatic mobilization of muscle, heart and lung is more often a curse. Unable to discharge through action the energy created, the response cannot run its course. The natural flow of events (running, fighting even killing) is not usually available to the civilized man. The response ability is all there and ready to go with no place to go. The process gets stuck and eventually the individual suffers from a condition known as sympatheticotonia, stuck and trapped in the Sympathetic response.

Muscles tighten, joints become stiff, the heart is continually stimulated in sympatheticotonia. Digestion becomes weak, the adrenal glands either keep the body constantly overcharged or else because of adrenal exhaustion the body becomes weak, tired and susceptible to inflammation and disease. Anxiety and distress become our constant companions.

Sympatheticotonia suggests that some or all of our 47 ganglia alongside of our spine have gone on and have stayed on. Overcoming stress and its effects must then really include an understanding of the structure of the Sympathetic nervous system and then an attempt to shut off or at least greatly diminish the action of the 2 gangliated cords of nerves that lie on either side of our spinal column. Any approach to stress reduction and relaxation should take into account the action and structure of our Sympathetic nervous system.

SCIENTIFIC RESEARCH

Some of the most interesting research on the function of the Sympathetic nervous system was done at the beginning of the 20th century by the noted Harvard physiologist, Dr. Walter Cannon. In his two books *Bodily Changes in Pain, Hunger, Fear and Rage* and also *The Wisdom of the Body* he explores every facet of what he calls the sympathetic-adrenal response.

One of his most interesting experiments consisted of the surgical removal of the gangliated cords from cats and dogs. These animals deprived of their Sympathetic nervous system continued to live, sometimes for years, after their operation. These animals survived quite well as long as they were not exposed to any undue stress like heat, cold or extreme physical exertion. When exposed to stress these surgically altered animals could not make the necessary internal adjustments to long survive.

The Sympathetic ganglia are not absolutely necessary for life but to maintain the homeostasis or internal balance of the organism under any kind of stress they are necessary. Only in the most secure and stress free environments do animals without their Sympathetic ganglia survive.

THE MESSAGE OF DISEASE

In many ways civilized man has created for himself just such an environment. Our clothing and central heating maintains a steady comfortable temperature; food is often plentiful and easy to obtain. The threat of attack from other creatures bent on catching us and eating us is mostly a thing of the past. In many ways we no longer need the presence of those 47 ganglia to mobilize and protect us from a dangerous environment. Although the need has passed, and only in the last 10 or 15 thousand years of human existence, we are still fully equipped to meet such emergencies. At some point in human history (probably within the last 10 or 15 thousand years) the 47 ganglia of our Sympathetic nervous system began to act on our bodies in a very different kind of way. Instead of being part of our necessary equipment in times of stress they have become our stress. The message of arousal, increased muscle tone and mobilization of energy has become for many of us constant anxiety, chronic tension and an inability to rest and relax.

OUR NATURAL STRENGTH AND HEALTH

Other physiological research conducted at the beginning of this century points to another interesting biological conclusion. Human cells given sufficient nutrition, the proper temperature and adequate waste removal will apparently live forever. Given an ideal environment, on a cellular level, we are immortal. Similarly, research done on the margin of safety to be found in the function of most of our organs has shown a huge, surplus capacity beyond what is necessary to sustain life.

Our cells, tissues and organs then have a resiliency and power beyond what we ordinarily need to survive. We are not frail and disease-prone creatures. Our natural endowments should, barring accidents, guarantee us health and very long life. Inasmuch as this is not usually the case, we may assume that something is impairing our smooth and healthy functioning.

BALANCE OF OUR INTERNAL ENVIRONMENT

Fatigue leads to breakdown and disease. Given the proper environment and nutrition, our cells, tissues and organs should remain healthy for 100 years or better. In searching for those agents that may be impairing our ability to maintain a balanced internal environment, we must come to those 47 ganglia of our Sympathetic nervous system. As long as any one of these stress messengers remains active, the muscles, organs and glands that receive stimulation from these ganglia will not be allowed their necessary rest. Only when Sympathetic stimulation diminishes can the Parasympathetic bring peace, rest and recuperation into the affected area.

Too many of us find ourselves permanently in the grip of Sympathetic function. Large areas of our bodies are under the constant influence of Sympathetic ganglia, and we are ripe there for breakdown and disease. Release this area, in time, from the grip of Sympathetic stimulation and it will quickly repair and grow strong and healthy again.

CHIROPRACTICS AND OSTEOPATHY

Certain unorthodox branches of the practice of medicine address themselves to this condition of chronic Sympathetic stimulation. Within the last 100 years both Chiropractics and Osteopathy have grown into respected and legitimate medical practices. Orthodox medicine has been reluctant to accept their legitimacy because of the weakness of the underlying theories they are based on. Manipulative therapies work and help people but the reason why they work has never been satisfactorily presented by the Chiropractic or Osteopathic profession.

Most manipulative therapies concentrate on the condition of the spinal column. Osteopaths see "lesions" of the column while Chiropractors treat what they call "subluxations". It is reasonable to assume that they are both seeing various anomalies and distortions in the structure of the spinal column. Their practice is based on correcting as much as possible those distortions and so bring the patient back into balance and health. Such an approach often works and not only to alleviate muscular and joint problems but also internal organ disturbances.

YOGA AND ACUPRESSURE

On the other side of the world in India and China an awareness and appreciation of the condition of the spine has been part of their medical and spiritual practices for thousands of years. In the more advanced practices of yoga a series of 6 or more chakras or centers in the spine are opened up and freed. With each chakra opened, the practitioner grows stronger and more healthy. The lower centers are usually freed first before the heart, throat and head centers are opened, but this is not always the case.

In Chinese medicine and health practice some of the centers they observe in the spine are considered so important as to be given names like "Door of Life", the kidney-associated center between the second and third lumbar vertebrae, and "Path of God", the heart-associated center between the fifth and sixth thoracic vertebrae.

On either side of the spine about one or two inches away from the center line of the back and in the muscular tissue lie a series of pressure points that are also organ related. These points are closely associated with internal organ function and both diagnoses and treatment consist in pressing those points to discover tenderness and to eventually alleviate that tenderness. Such treatments are not given simply to alleviate backache and muscular tension but also to help heal internal organs. Like Chiropractics and Osteopathy, the theories behind such treatments vary considerably but this does not diminish the fact that such treatments are often very effective.

47 MESSENGERS

It is a little surprising that with our current anatomical knowledge the most obvious conclusion has not been more clearly made and presented. Yes, there are distinct centers of nervous activity closely associated with the spine; these are the 47 ganglia of our Sympathetic nervous system. Yes, these centers both powerfully affect internal organs and also the level of tone (tension) in the muscular system. Even the most conventional and orthodox of modern physicians would concede these facts.

It has been left up to the manipulative therapists to make practical use of these anatomical facts. Yet the exact nature of the healing process that Chiropractors, Osteopaths and other manipulators are engaged in has not been clearly demonstrated. This may be the case because a crucial (perhaps the crucial) element in such treatments is often absent and not even mentioned. That element is rest.

THE NEED FOR REST

Manipulative therapies are simply based on a mechanical model of understanding the body. If a part is bad, if you can even see that it is bad (the lesions and subluxations of the spinal vertebrae), then fix it and the device will work better.

Yet if we begin to look a little further and a little deeper we discover a kind of devil at work beneath the problem we can see and treat. That devil is Sympatheticotonia or an overactivity of the Sympathetic ganglia. All our efforts at cure and correction are really for that end. Diminish the activity of the ganglia and release the person from the grip of his distress. And although all manipulations and adjustments are moving in that direction, the actual goal of release happens during moments of stillness and rest.

Eastern medicine has not lost sight of this fact. Meditation, inner awareness and deepening relaxation has always been an important part of their health practices. It is here we come up against the real paradox in healing. The easiest thing to do in the world is nothing; being still, letting go and relaxing. Yet for creatures bedeviled by a particular part of their nervous system into perpetual activity, arousal and agitation, it is nearly impossible. Sick people cannot rest. They are stuck in a primitive response that has probably caused their disease in the first place and is now keeping them from getting the rest, the deep release and relaxation, that would be their cure.

In this sense Chiropractors, Osteopaths and manipulators are trying to induce a natural, healing state of rest and release into the afflicted part of the body and also into the person as a whole. Rest is foreign to many of us. We do not like to do it because we think nothing is achieved when we rest and we must always be achieving, be doing something. Our culture seems to demand and expect this kind of constant drive from people. We seem to accept rest and relaxation only in those we call retired.

Retiring is what most of us need to do right now. The idea that we should at frequent intervals in our lives retire and seek stillness, rest and release from tension can save our lives and prolong them. By recognizing that we are bedeviled by 47 distinct nerve centers that deliver a message of arousal, tension and eventually disease, we can conceive of a means to end our diseases.

TURNING OFF SYMPATHETIC GANGLIA

Let us conclude with an example of just such an approach. Perhaps the most important and active of all the ganglia is a pair called the superior cervical ganglia. This is the top pair of ganglion on the gangliated cords lying in close proximity to the second and third cervical vertebrae at the very top of the neck. These ganglia have nerve branches accompanying blood vessels into the head and brain. Other branches go to the eyes and to the mucous membranes of the nose and mouth. Still more nerve branches emerge from these ganglia and go to the throat and heart. Disturbances in any of these areas should be traced back to the activity of the superior cervical ganglia. The continual action of this one pair of ganglion precludes the possibility of the head, throat and heart of ever getting sufficient rest and relaxation for their proper and healthy functioning. Also because these ganglia lie at the very top of the gangliated cords, they have a large role to play in turning on the rest of the Sympathetic system and thereby stressing the entire body.

Turning off these Sympathetic nerve bulbs requires becoming aware of the tension and stiffness at the top of the spine. Recurring areas of stiffness in the spine suggest Sympathetic ganglia have turned on and resist going off. Manipulation and adjustment of the spine and the muscles near it sets the process of relaxation and release into motion. Applying pressure to the area of the superior cervical ganglia has a relaxing and restorative effect on the head, throat and heart. As this important nerve center releases during periods of rest, the effects may even radiate throughout the body.

THE STRESS WHEEL

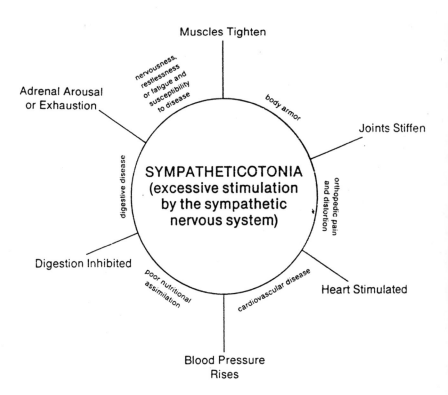

REFERENCES

CONFESSIONS OF A KNIFE, Richard Selzer, M.D., Simon and Schuster, 1979.

GRAY'S ANATOMY, Henry Gray, Crown Publishers, 1977.

BODILY CHANGES IN PAIN, HUNGER, FEAR AND RAGE, Walter Cannon, M.D., Charles T. Branford Co., 1953.

THE WISDOM OF THE BODY, Walter Cannon, M.D., W.W. Norton and Co., 1932.

MAN IN THE TRAP, Elsworth F. Baker, M.D., Avon Books, 1967.

POSTURAL RELATIONS TO THE AUTONOMIC NERVOUS SYSTEM, Thomas M. Parker, D.C., Health research, 1963.

BREATH, SLEEP, THE HEART AND LIFE, Pundit Acharya, Dawn Horse Press, 1975.

AWAKEN HEALING ENERGY THROUGH THE TAO, Mantak Chia, Copen Press, 1981.

DO-IT-YOURSELF SHIATSU, Wataru Ohashi, E.P. Dutton and Co., 1976.

AQUARIAN AGE HEALING, John Hurley, D.C. and Helen Saunders, D.C., Health Research, 1963.

OSTEOPATHIC MEDICINE, AN AMERICAN REFORMATION, George Northup, D.O., American Osteopathic Association, 1966.

TYPE A BEHAVIOR AND YOUR HEART, Meyer Friedman, M.D., and Ray H. Rosenman, M.D., Ballantine Books, 1974.

CHIROTHERAPY, Phillips DeHesse, Health Research, 1974.

UNDER THE INFLUENCE OF ADRENALIN

UNDER THE INFLUENCE OF ADRENALIN

Of all the hormones that the body naturally produces, none is more quick acting or as dramatic in its effect as adrenalin. Adrenalin is the emergency hormone that prepares the body for what has come to be known as the "fight or flight" response. During times of stress adrenalin is literally squirted into our blood stream by the inner section of the adrenal glands, that part of the gland called the adrenal medulla. Unlike the secretions of the outer part of the gland, the cortex, adrenalin is not essential for life. The various steroid hormones produced by the cortex, including cortisone and the mineralcorticoids, are indeed essential for the maintenance of life.

Although adrenalin may not be essential for life, it certainly has played an important role in the survival of animals on our planet. Adrenalin gives strength and power; it prepares animals and man for the struggle for existence. It increases the beat and power of the heart. It redirects the nourishing blood flow away from internal organs and into the muscles and brain. It increases energy by inducing the liver to release glucose into the blood. Adrenalin arouses and stimulates the body into action.

Adrenalin is nerve juice. The adrenal medulla is actually a large concentration of nerve cells that grow in the embryo out of the same tissue that also becomes our sympathetic nervous system. In fact the sympathetic nervous system and the secretion of adrenalin into the blood have almost identical effects on the body. Sympathetic nerves secrete at their nerve endings a neurotransmitter chemical very similar to adrenalin. Where the sympathetic nervous system acts by minute secretions of this adrenalin-like chemical at specific nerve endings, the adrenal medulla, the inner part of the adrenal gland, literally pours this potent nerve juice directly into the blood stream.

Adrenalin acts as a powerful and more sustaining back up to the action of the sympathetic nerves. Both the sympathetic nervous system and the presence of adrenalin in the blood act to stimulate, tone and arouse the body. Adrenalin's effect is more long lasting and sustained than the action of the sympathetic nerves alone. Acting together they form the sympathetic-adrenal system and it is this system that is the body's most immediate and dramatic call to action.

For countless millions of years man and animals have relied on this autonomic mobilization of energy, strength, speed and power to escape enemies or to catch food. Without this sympathetic-adrenal system animals in the natural state could not long survive. Only within the last ten or fifteen thousand years has man started to outgrow his need for this very ancient biological system. Although civilized man may not really need the physical prowess that the sympathetic-adrenal system provides, he is still fully equipped with this autonomic system of arousal.

Civilized men and women are no doubt still deeply affected by the presence and action of the sympathetic-adrenal system. What we admire as drive, ambition, intellectual sharpness, willpower and determination in people may be largely due to the increased tone and energy that the sympathetic-adrenal creates. Can the achievements and wealth of our modern, technological world be explained simply by the fact that man is a very intelligent animal? It is probably more accurate to say that man is a very intelligent animal with a lot of drive. Without drive and determination our intelligence does not amount to much. Our capacity for sustained and collective efforts has had as much to do with our success as our intelligence.

Success has its price; our drive takes its toll. Arousal in the natural state usually runs it course. Arousal in civilized men and women rarely does. Some level of almost constant arousal may even be a necessary prerequisite to civilized functioning. To work, to pursue long range goals, to sustain a constant and daily effort as most people must do requires some level of steady arousal and mobilization of energy. This degree of arousal may make us materially successful but eventually it will leave us physically and spiritually exhausted. Real relaxation becomes difficult if not impossible. Peace, inner harmony and an ability to rest are virtually unattainable. We find ourselves surrounded by almost unimaginable wealth, comfort and technological achievements but peace and simple pleasure elude us. Even our creations come to enslave us. How many of us are slaves to the telephone, automobile and television?

LIMITING AROUSAL

The world's major religions all had their beginnings in a quest to find inner harmony and balance. Our contemporary knowledge of the functioning of the sympathetic-adrenal system gives us, perhaps, an extra edge in understanding the nature of our distress and giving us a course to relieve it.

This course is a conscious program of limiting arousal. The hundreds of techniques of relaxation and meditation move us in that direction. We consciously begin to disengage ourselves from enslavement to the instruments that perpetuate our arousal and restlessness. These instruments may be anything from the TV set to the hum and buzz of our own thoughts. They all conspire to keep us busy and aroused. Whole lives can be spent running from and avoiding the simple need to rest.

Unfortunately, rest does not come easy. It is as if some invisible hand has gripped us from behind and impels us to keep moving. There may be a glimmer of realization that we should stop and rest but the compulsion to move and do forces us on. We hear the cracking of the whip over our heads every waking moment of our lives, and although we may be running on empty we can't stop running.

BETWEEN THE BLADES: PATH OF GOD

From an area between our shoulder blades in back arise the nerves that stimulate the secretion of adrenalin. This crucial nerve center between the blades has been called "Path of God" in the native Chinese mystical tradition of Taoism. Early on the Chinese realized that the opening of this center had a profound effect not only on our hearts but on our spiritual being as well. Open the center between the blades and turn off the adrenalin spigot. Release, align and soften between the blades and find the possibility of quiet and peace within yourself.

Many of us have hardened and toughened between the blades in back. A year or ten may not be enough to undo the damage we have done to ourselves. Yet to know about this center and to begin its release is to be on the "Path of God".

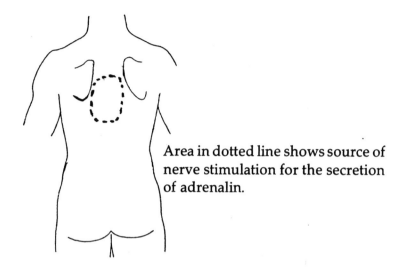

Area in dotted line shows source of nerve stimulation for the secretion of adrenalin.

REFERENCES

GRAY'S ANATOMY, Henry Gray, Crown Publishers, 1977.

BODILY CHANGES IN PAIN, HUNGER, FEAR AND RAGE, Walter Cannon, M.D., Charles T. Branford Co., 1953.

THE WISDOM OF THE BODY, Walter Cannon, M.D., W.W. Norton and Co., 1932.

POSTURAL RELATIONS TO THE AUTONOMIC NERVOUS SYSTEM, Thomas M. Parker, D.C., Health research, 1963.

BREATH, SLEEP, THE HEART AND LIFE, Pundit Acharya, Dawn Horse Press, 1975.

TYPE A BEHAVIOR AND YOUR HEART, Meyer Friedman, M.D., and Ray H. Rosenman, M.D., Ballantine Books, 1974.

DO-IT-YOURSELF SHIATSU, Wataru Ohashi, E.P. Dutton and Co., 1976.

THE STRESS OF LIFE, Hans Selye, M.D., McGraw Hill, 1976.

THE SABBATH, Abraham Joshua Heschel, Farrar, Straus and Giroux, 1951.

DAY
OF
REST

DAY OF REST

Without leaving his door
He knows everything under heaven.
Without looking out of his window
He knows all the ways of heaven.
For the further one travels
The less one knows.
Therefore the Sage arrives without going,
Sees all without looking,
Does nothing, yet achieves everything.

from the TAO TE CHING
translation by Arthur Waley

The ancient Jews took their Sabbath seriously. Those who did not keep the Sabbath were sometimes stoned to death. Ever since man felt the need to put in a week of work, he has probably felt the need to rest a day once in awhile. Out of this felt need to rest must have come the holy day of the Sabbath, a day set aside not only for rest and relaxation but also for worship and contemplation.

Anthropologists have found that many primitive societies are not always as brutish and hard as we would like to think. Some still surviving gathering-hunting peoples rest and play as much or more than they work. This fact throws a curious new light on civilization. What good is civilization if it means more toil?

Actually civilization does not necessarily mean less work; it means more security. Civilization is a struggle with the forces of nature. It is an attempt to secure food and shelter and a lifestyle somewhat safe from the vagaries and hardships that a life in nature can mean. Very few of us could or would want to return to a life in nature. We have sacrificed a more natural and at-ease part of ourselves to become civilized, but we have gained comfort, security and a more stimulating existence.

The fact remains that many people even in this year of 1980 work around forty hours a week, five days a week. Most of us lead regimented lives that require for eight hours a day we comply to a schedule that may not fit us. We may want to sleep, but we must work. We may feel like walking, but we have to sit. We may be hungry but cannot eat. We may even be sick and tired, but we continue to work.

The demands of life require that we maintain ourselves for the better part of our days at some level of activity. Our lives can be divided into two basic levels of functioning. One of these levels is characterized by activity and stimulation and one by inactivity and rest. These two basic modes of existence can also be understood in terms of our autonomic nervous system as the sympathetic and parasympathetic respectively.

Our autonomic nervous system is sometimes referred to as our vegetative nervous system because it is the oldest and most primitive component of our nervous system. Before all the complexities of higher brain centers developed through evolution, creatures had an autonomic system regulating internal function and the cycles of life.

In *The Dragons of Eden* Carl Sagan discusses how the evolution of nerve tissue took place by the addition of further sophisticated and complex structures but not by the elimination of the older, more primitive ones. He describes our autonomic and forebrain structures as essentially reptillian in their construction. On top of this reptillian brain and nervous system, we have added our human apparatus for thinking, controlling and doing. This is a simplistic explanation of nervous system evolution but essentially adequate for purposes here.

On the most fundamental level our functioning is divided into two parts: activity and stimulation (sympathetic function) and inactivity and rest (parasympathetic function). An abundance of information has appeared on stress and sympathetic activity. Only rather recently have scientists and doctors turned their attention from stress reactions to our innate capacity to rest and relax. Dr. Herbert Benson's book, *The Relaxation*

Response, is one of the few books to address itself to the question of parasympathetic function in a scientific way and at that it is a tentative and incomplete picture. Dr. Benson's conclusion seems to be that deep rest for twenty minutes twice a day is what we need and too much more than that can be harmful and even dangerous to one's mental stability. One also gets the impression that we rest so we can go back to work and not that we work so we can eventually rest. Western science and technology are the products of work and activity. Science comes from stimulation, curiosity, experimentation, thinking and activity. No doubt in its first few glimpses into another side of life it will see something threatening and disruptive.

ANOTHER SIDE TO LIFE

Who knows how to rest now-a-days? Weekends mean a ride in the car, going shopping, playing sports, parties, drinking and eating. This is fine and a welcome change from the work week but where is the time for doing nothing, letting go, rest and relaxation? What has happened to a day devoted to quietness and rest? Where is that day set aside for the body and spirit to heal and recover, a time to grow heavy and tired, to feel our weariness into our muscles and joints and to allow the healing currents in rest and relaxation to make us new and better. We have forgotten our bodies and ignore this other side of life.

For many of us it takes a sickness to slow us down enough to rest. Giving oneself a day a week or even a day every other week to do nothing but rest and heal has been part of our culture for thousands of years. This is the Sabbath, a holy day of rest, a day that is little observed anymore.

THE PARASYMPATHETIC RESPONSE

Devoting an entire day or the better part of a day to relaxation and rest allows for the unfolding of a particular process that can be called the parasympathetic response. The parasympathetic response acts as a balance for our otherwise active and creative lives. In fact, our continued ability to perform and work depends equally on our ability to relax and to rest. Of course, sleep is our most common and frequent rest but often in the course of our lives we need something more. This something more is the parasympathetic response.

The parasympathetic response goes beyond the relaxation response elucidated by Dr. Benson in his book of the same name. Dr. Benson sees the relaxation response as an innate potential in all bodies to slow down and relax. One only needs to have some peace and quiet, a comfortable place to sit or lie down, and possibly a mental object to focus the mind on. Very important, though, is maintaining a passive attitude towards what may take place. Trying too hard to relax is self-defeating. If the ego cannot let go even a little and allow the process to happen, no real relaxation can take place.

Unfortunately Dr. Benson believes that this process is best confined to two twenty minute periods twice a day. He hasn't seen the truth to a larger and deeper sense of the relaxation response; that for the process to really blossom may take a day, sometimes more. The weariness, the exhaustion, the accumulation of physical tension that happens to all of us in our work, our play and our relationships takes its heavy toll. If twenty minutes twice a day were only enough; for most of us the real healing and rejuvenating process of rest and relaxation often requires a day or better. Perhaps we cannot find the pure and open time to do absolutely nothing in every week of our lives, but fifteen or twenty times a year we need to rest and relax for a day.

RELAXATION AND THE KINESTHETIC SENSE

Some people can greatly relax in a short period of time. Yet for most of us relaxation does not come that easy. Most of our tension is real and persistent. It has become part of our character and personality. To learn to relax completely takes years and usually requires the practice of special exercises and the application of deep massage to the locked regions of muscles and tendons where our tensions live. Let us just say that we will not learn to completely relax in a day or week or even in a year. What we can do in a shorter period of time is become aware of our tension and our fatigue.

Ironically we need to relax a little to feel how tense and tired we are. A deeper sense of ourselves, a sense that goes into the muscles and joints, is called kinesthesia. Sensory nerves deep into our muscles and joints relay to the brain our inner condition. Yet for this inner sense to break into our consciousness requires a calming of that consciousness. A mind always busy and turned out towards worldly affairs cannot see or feel the internal state of affairs. The kinesthetic sense is subtle and usually all but lost in the din and spectacle of sights, sounds, and active thought.

The human species is singularly adept at ignoring and suppressing its physical needs for rest and relaxation.

Western civilization, especially, has maintained an outward and active approach to living. We enjoy a high level of stimulation and have created an interesting and exciting world. Our achievements, though, have their cost. The tranquilizer, Valium, is the most prescribed drug in the United States. Great achievement often means high levels of activity and stimulation (sympathetic function). At some point our levels of excitement and stimulation can overwhelm us. We cannot sit still or find any peace and comfort. Our nerves feel jangled and frayed. We become jumpy and irritable; we are probably very tired but hardly know it because of our constant and high level of excitement. Our perpetual desire to do, to make, to go disinclines us towards any real repose and rest.

Now the body has its own built in tranquilizing system, the parasympathetic half of our autonomic nervous system. Unlike most other aspects of life, to enjoy real rest one must practice inactivity. Doing nothing is an art in that it is allowing nature, one's own physical nature, to have its way with us. Doing nothing does not mean that nothing happens. Doing nothings allows for the emergence of our fatigue and an awareness of our tension and stiffness. Doing nothing allows a long denied and sorely needed respite from excitement and stimulation to unfold.

Practicing passivity can mean a return to equilibrium for many of us. Our egos know very well how to grasp and hold on. To rest one must begin to loosen the ego's grasping sense on life. We are all blocked and stiff, resisting a powerful inner current of life and energy that could heal and nourish us.

Trying to elicit the parasympathetic response involves time and waiting. Maintaining a passive attitude and keeping relatively still and physically comfortable are prerequisites. Perhaps nothing will begin to happen in twenty minutes or twenty hours, but usually a few hours is enough to allow the resting response to begin functioning.

How many of us are running away from some inner reality! As the resting state deepens and we begin to feel our accumulated tensions and dis-ease, we will want to run away. Do not be afraid; let the repose and stillness deepen further. Feel how tired you have become, be aware of the fatigue. Allow yourself to feel the aches and pains of tension and stiffness. Thoughts may revolt, churn, get nasty and insist that you get up and do something. Let them happen and continue to relax, be still, let go and rest. There is nothing you must do that cannot wait.

You may sense a heaviness develop in the limbs and body. Your muscles are beginning to give up their struggle and are softening and relaxing. Allow the heavy feeling to have its way with you. Be heavy, immovable, weigh a thousand pounds. The world is not crashing down around you; you are finding your center. Let it happen.

Do you feel like stretching a little or revolving a joint through a range of motion? Go ahead. Here you are feeling and responding to a natural need for a natural kind of exercise. Slowly stretching muscles and gently moving parts of your body are easy and therapeutic and can be an integral part of a day of rest.

Getting into a hot tub and soaking for an hour also fits nicely into a resting day's routine. Don't take a magazine to read. Just lay back and soak. The hot water will soften and loosen your muscular tissue. Feel the tensions and stiffnesses that have accumulated throughout your body release and melt away.

A SOFT BODY

People are generally misguided into thinking that being hard is the desired physical state to achieve. Hardness in a muscle means that muscle is tense. A hard body is one in a state of contraction. Chronic hardness in any part of the musculature means that the flow of internal fluids and feelings are blocked there. Hardness implies being closed off or deadened in that area. As long as one consciously or unconsciously fears the process of softening and loosening there can be little real rest.

Rest requires some state of relaxation of muscles. Relaxing muscles has a sense of opening and expanding to it. There is a release and a letting go and often a feeling of relief as some area, chronically held tight, lets go and relaxes. The area will become softer and will feel more like liquid encased in skin. In fact our bodies are essentially made up of seventy percent water. Water is our essential nature and as we learn to relax and return to a more natural style of life, we can feel how watery we are. Our muscles feel like water, we move like water, we find a sense of ease and flow. Hard muscles and hard bodies struggle and fight with life and generally deny and destroy nature as they find it outside themselves and within. Softness is tolerant and yielding. It isn't weakness but intelligence and maturity to learn to be a part of the world and to move to its rhythms and flows.

REST AND RELIGIOUS EXPERIENCE

As rest and relaxation evolve over a day or over longer periods of time, the mind and body begin to slow down. Time will no longer seem to be pressing down on us demanding achievement and purpose. Breathing deepens down into the belly. The mind sinks, and the internal racket of incessant thought begins to quiet down. Our senses become purified and open, and for a little while we are simple and uncomplicated creatures again.

Almost every sacred tradition glorifies rest and relaxation as ways to spiritual experience. God does not reside in heaven above or earth below so much as within our own nature. We cannot grasp religious feeling, we can only allow it to happen. Rest and relaxation are a form of worship. Resting can open a door to peace and quietude. As rest and relaxation deepen and fulfill their natural function, we become centered and still. The natural world impresses us. A sense of beauty pervades and surrounds us. A quiet pleasure holds us gently.

The wind may carry us away. The sound of leaves rustling is rapturous music. Beauty and peace are everywhere. The belly, the heart, the head open and release the aches that live there. We are free and in the hands of God.

REFERENCES

ORIGINS, Richard Leakey, E.P. Dutton, 1977.

THE WAY AND ITS POWER, A STUDY OF THE TAO TE CHING, Arthur Waley, Grove Press, 1958.

DRAGONS OF EDEN, Carl Sagan, Ballantine Book, 1977.

THE RELAXATION RESPONSE, Dr. Herbert Benson, William Morrow & Co., 1975.

BIOENERGETICS, Dr. Alexander Lowen, Penguin Books, 1975.

THE WATERCOURSE WAY, Alan Watts, Pantheon Books, 1975.

RESURRECTION OF THE BODY, F. Matthias Alexander, Delta Book, 1974.

THE SABBATH, Abraham Joshua Heschel, Farrar, Straus and Giroux, 1951.

MIND AS HEALER, MIND AS SLAYER, Kenneth R. Pelletier, Delta, 1977.

THE SCIENCE OF RELIGION, Paramahansa Yogananda, Self-Realization Fellowship, 1953.